"In Kim Henry's warm and gracious ~~~ those of us who may think our best years are behind us ~~ 'Wait. You matter, even now and especially now. Your prayers matter. Your talents matter. Your perspective matters.' What sweet affirmation. What nourishment for the soul. Using Scripture, godly wisdom, quotes from Christian leaders, and heartfelt prayers, Kim takes us on a journey to understand how valuable we truly are. Especially to God. Please read *Do I Still Matter?* and rejoice in this time of your life."

—**Jeanette Levellie**, author of *Hello, Beautiful! Finally Love Yourself Just As You Are*

"*Do I Still Matter?* tenderly penetrates the depths of an aging soul with a resounding *Yes!* Just when you thought the world had sidelined you, Kim Henry uses God's Word to shift your perspective and remind you that with age comes incredible benefits that truly matter to God and His kingdom."

—**Lisa Martin**, women's speaker, Lisa Martin Ministries

"'Do I still matter' is a question people ask at any age, but especially as we grow older and begin to see ourselves through the lens of a younger generation. While we may feel like we've got storehouses full of wisdom and experience as we age, others often view us as outdated and irrelevant. Kim Henry's book nails this burning question with God's divine truth and perspective. Her devotional format is a perfect way to receive daily encouragement from the Word. Every chapter is filled with Scripture, prayer, and a secret key to growing older with confidence in the person God made us to be . . . at any age. Enjoy!"

—**Dr. Mary Ann Noack**, pastor of women's ministries, River West Church, Lake Oswego, Oregon

"Kim Henry has addressed the unexpected situations we find ourselves in as we grow older. I faced this dilemma at the age of fifty when I was laid off from my job of twenty-five years. After a merger, the layoff wasn't unexpected, since many others lost their jobs in the takeover too. However, the surprise was that it was difficult to find another job with all my experience. . . . I prayed daily for God to show me where He wanted me. But the months of waiting with no job made me ask God if He was done with me. Was I no longer important? Did I still matter? . . . In this thorough book, the author covers all the thoughts and questions we have as we age, and affirms that God has the answers to all of them. I highly recommend this book for anyone who is facing the challenges of age, and how to handle those challenges in a positive way, the way God would have us do."

—**Marilyn Turk**, award-winning author of
more than twenty books and novellas

DO

I

STILL

MATTER?

The Secrets of Aging
with FAITH and PURPOSE

KIM TAYLOR HENRY

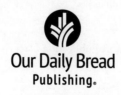

Our Daily Bread
Publishing.

Do I Still Matter? The Secrets of Aging with Faith and Purpose
© 2024 by Kimberly Taylor Henry

Requests for permission to quote from this book should be directed to: Permissions Department, Our Daily Bread Publishing, PO Box 3566, Grand Rapids, MI 49501, or contact us by email at permissionsdept@odb.org.

Scripture quotations, unless otherwise indicated, are taken from the *Holy Bible*, New Living Translation, copyright © 1996, 2004, 2015 by Tyndale House Foundation. Used by permission of Tyndale House Publishers, Carol Stream, Illinois 60188. All rights reserved.
    Scripture quotations marked CEV are from the Contemporary English Version. Copyright © 1991, 1992, 1995 by American Bible Society. Used by permission.
    Scripture quotations marked MSG are taken from *The Message*, copyright © 1993, 2002, 2018 by Eugene H. Peterson. Used by permission of NavPress. All rights reserved. Represented by Tyndale House Publishers.
    Scripture quotations marked NIV are taken from the Holy Bible, New International Version®, NIV®. Copyright © 1973, 1978, 1984, 2011 by Biblica, Inc.™ Used by permission of Zondervan. All rights reserved worldwide. www.zondervan.com.

Interior design by Michael J. Williams

ISBN: 978-1-64070-332-2

Library of Congress Cataloging-in-Publication Data Available

Printed in China
25 26 27 28 29 30 31 / 8 7 6 5 4 3 2

Contents

Introduction
Doubt Creeps In

I didn't want her to believe me.

I had just turned fifty-five years old and was now eligible for an "age fifty-five-plus" discount. I felt certain that when I requested it, the cashier would look aghast and exclaim, "You couldn't possibly be that old! May I see your ID?" But no, she merely said, "Okay, that'll be $23.15 then."

"Don't you want to see some ID?"

"No." She bagged my purchase. "No one's going to claim to be a senior citizen if they're not."

She had a point there. Still, the experience left my confidence shaken. Was I really a senior citizen? Was this the beginning of the end?

No, but it was a beginning, the beginning of a new chapter in my life, one that was going to take some getting used to.

***

Fast (startlingly fast) forward. Years have passed, and I look back on that "am I really a senior citizen?" moment and laugh. Fifty-five had felt so old. It now sounds young. Yes, "senior citizen" status took getting used to. I balked and bucked for a while, like a horse getting used to a saddle. And yes, it has been and still is quite a ride. But I'm more comfortable in it now. I no longer bristle at the thought that I don't have the energy level of my children and grandchildren.

I'm (almost) getting used to the fact that my face and body aren't the same as they used to be. I've learned to appreciate and enjoy the wisdom, luxuries of time, and other bonuses being a "senior" brings. My questions of whether I still matter have been answered. I do! And in many ways. Not exactly the same ones as when I was younger, but beautiful, valuable, and significant nonetheless.

The senior chapter in life has two paths from which to choose. Satan's path is wide open and easily accessible. But it is a way of discouragement, sadness, lamenting, and languishing. God's path is one of joy, adventure, and flourishing. Thankfully, as Christians, we can readily walk that path by faith, fulfilling God's purpose for us and discovering the secrets to a life stage of opportunities and delights. The goal is to internalize and live those secrets. Together, let's explore what a gift this chapter of life can be.

—Kim Taylor Henry

1

The Question Forms

My days are swifter than a runner. . . .
They skim past like boats of papyrus.
Job 9:25–26 NIV

When we're young, we'd like to be older; days fly, years inch along. When we're older, we'd like to be younger; days can seem long, years whiz by. The seemingly slow passage of time we experience as youths eager to grow up topsy-turveys into a rapid blur of passing years.

I'm the baby of our family. I have only one sister. She is nearly seven years older than me. Growing up, she never let me forget it. She flaunted her privileges and perceived wisdom of years. As we got older, the tables turned. I felt no guilt reminding her of her age. My "baby" status became a delight for me. But gradually, insidiously, the signs began. I felt stiff after sitting. My hands resembled my mother's. Was that a new wrinkle in my cheek, or did I just sleep on my face? Why was I yawning by 9:00 p.m.?

"Inside this body there's an eighteen-year-old wondering what in the world happened." That about summed it up. My chronological age and the age I saw myself at were growing further apart. I balked at my newfound understanding of "old people" jokes.

My childhood aims were to please my parents, do well in school, have a successful career and happy marriage, and create a family. As a child, I was the apple of my parents' eyes. When I met my future husband, I was his desire. In my career, my input was valued, sought out. I had three children and was the center of their universe. During my entire life, I had mattered—to my parents, my husband, my children, my job, and more. I'd felt focused, productive, needed, valuable.

Then, bit by bit, my importance diminished. At least, that's how it seemed. My parents went to heaven. School was a distant memory. My career concluded. My marriage lost the passion of youth. Many of my accomplishments were behind me. My children left home to pursue lives of their own. Parents with children looked too young to have them. Their worlds were full speed ahead. The pace of mine had slowed. I'd always felt involved and valued. Suddenly I wasn't so sure. I began to ask God, "Do I still matter?"

Dear God,

Sometimes I'm overwhelmed by time's passage. It rushes by like raging wind. I used to see the age I'm at as old. Now that I'm here, I don't feel old. It's a different view from this perspective. I'm still me, with so much to offer. My fear is that no one will want it. I want to still matter, Lord. I need my life to have purpose. Show me how to remain valuable and vital. It seems like just yesterday I had it all ahead of me. Now much of what I looked forward to is in the past. When I stood at the threshold of my life, I had no knowledge of what it would be like, who I'd become, where I'd live, what I'd do, or with whom I'd do it. Now I know. I've lived it. Looking back, what I see is the major portion of the years I'll have on this earth. Yet with your grace, I have many years to look forward to. Show me I still matter. Amen.

SECRET #1

God's way opens the door to a new life stage of opportunities and delights.

2

My Focus on Others Matters

*Anyone who wants to be first must be the
very last, and the servant of all.*

Mark 9:35 NIV

"Do I still matter?" is a normal, natural concern. Yet the more attention we give that question, the further we stray from its answer. Asking it is focusing on ourselves rather than on others. The Bible tells us to do the opposite.

> Don't be selfish; don't try to impress others. . . . Don't look out only for your own interests, but take an interest in others, too. (Philippians 2:3–4)

> **Lord, grant that I might not so much seek . . . to be loved as to love.** PRAYER OF SAINT FRANCIS

If we focus on showing others they matter, we'll find life's greatest blessings, and we'll matter greatly.

No one enjoys someone who's self-absorbed. Self-absorption does not bring happiness. King Solomon had great riches and the ability to pursue whatever he chose. Yet in the book of Ecclesiastes he described life as "meaningless" thirty times in twelve short chapters. Could that have been due, in part, to his self-focus? For in those chapters he used *I, me* or *myself* over one hundred times.

The more we concentrate on showing others they matter instead of worrying whether we do, and the more we give of ourselves to them, the more we will matter.

> Give, and you will receive. Your gift will return to you in full—pressed down, shaken together to make room for more, running over, and poured into your lap. The amount you give will determine the amount you get back. (Luke 6:38)

While the point is not to care about others so they'll care about us, God did plant that bonus in this paradox. Jesus said, "If you cling to your life, you will lose it; but if you give up your life for me, you will find it" (Matthew 10:39). If we cling to concern about ourselves, we'll lose the full and abundant life Jesus offers.

Dear God,
Rescue me from worry over whether I matter. Help me end the foolishness of nursing wounds and mulling over others' opinions of me. May I stop thinking about what I'm getting and focus on what I'm giving. Guide me in putting my energy toward showing, by my words and actions, that you and others matter to me. Nudge me to share with others that they matter to you. May my motivation never be what's in it for me but only a desire to live as you've taught, love as you've loved, and serve you by serving others. Instead of asking myself what others are thinking of me, remind me to ask what I'm doing for them. Thank you for the gift that in meeting others' needs, my own needs are often met. Open my eyes to opportunities to serve without a thought to the cost or return. Fill my heart with such devotion to you and such concern for others that there's no room left to be concerned with whether I matter. Amen.

SECRET #2

If I focus on showing others they matter, I'll experience some of life's greatest blessings.

3

What the World Thinks Doesn't Matter

The wisdom of this world is foolishness to God.
1 Corinthians 3:19

It's no fun to feel left behind, blending in with the background, fading into unimportance, no longer critical at work, needed by our children, desired by our spouse. Because we live in a youth-enthralled culture, it's an easy, but erroneous, mindset to fall into. Advertising, beauty products, clothing, entertainment, athletics, employment, you name it, all scream "being young is where it's at."

God's Word tells us to not care what the world thinks. "Our purpose is to please God, not people" (1 Thessalonians 2:4). If we find ourselves sliding into a worldly view that youth is better than age, we can, with the apostle Paul, ask, "Am I now trying to win the approval of human beings, or of God?" (Galatians 1:10 NIV).

The world may reject the wisdom God has granted us through our experiences. We may identify with Proverbs 1:23–25:

> Come and listen to my counsel. I'll share my heart with you and make you wise. I called you so often, but you wouldn't come. I reached out to you, but you paid no attention. You ignored my advice and rejected the correction I offered.

But God values wisdom. He calls those who have gained it "blessed" (3:13 NIV).

> **Faith does not eliminate questions. But faith knows where to take them.**   ELIZABETH ELLIOT

God doesn't determine worth by age. He sees in terms of eternity. It's our beliefs, faith, actions, words, and attitudes that matter to him. He "does not look at the things people look at. People look at the outward appearance, but the LORD looks at the heart" (1 Samuel 16:7 NIV). Do you think he gives any thought to the fact that we're fifty-five, sixty-five, seventy-five or more years old? No, for he assures us "the godly will flourish. . . . Even in old age they will still produce fruit, they will remain vital and green" (Psalm 92:12, 14).

We can't and shouldn't isolate ourselves from the world, but we can live in the world but "not conform to the pattern of this world" (Romans 12:2 NIV). The closer our relationship with God, the more ageless we'll feel, and the more we'll understand we still matter. We can relax and enjoy the gifts this life stage has to offer. Instead of feeling washed out or washed up, we can wash in God's "river of delights" (Psalm 36:8). When we bring to God, rather than to the world, our questions of whether we still have worth, he will answer with a resounding "YES!"

Dear God,
I look to you, not the world, for my answers. Thank you that with you, age doesn't matter. Let it not matter to me either. Take my attention off my age and put it on who I am inside. I give you my heart. Guide me, use me, fill me with joy in you. May I be in this world but not conform to this world. Keep me on guard against the world's influencing me. I want to focus on pleasing you, not the world. Remind me that age measures only my time on this earth, not my worth. Help me to never give undue attention to the number of my years. Amen.

SECRET #3

God doesn't determine worth by age.

4

My Choice of
Perspective Matters

Turn your ears to wisdom, and
concentrate on understanding.

Proverbs 2:2

How we look at things impacts our life, and how we look at things is a choice. We can elect to (inaccurately) see this life stage as one in which we don't matter, or we can (accurately) see it as one in which we matter, just in different ways than we have before. We can spend our time bemoaning the loss of our former roles, or we can look forward to fresh accomplishments in new roles. We can fruitlessly wish time would stand still, or we can enjoy the ever-changing flow of life as planned by God.

Our perspective can be that this life chapter is one of opportunity as we open our eyes to each day's potential. "This is the day the LORD has made. [I] will rejoice and be glad in it" (Psalm 118:24). We have the time now to absorb, to contemplate, to fully engage.

> Each of us must take responsibility for our own attitude. If you want today to be a good day, you need to take charge of the way you look at it. JOHN MAXWELL

The perspective we choose will make the difference between our feeling doleful and our feeling soul-full. We can lament gray hair, or we can look on it as the Bible does—"a crown of splendor . . .

attained in the way of righteousness" (Proverbs 16:31 NIV). We can fall into a pit of self-pity, or we can realize that all of life is a gift to be fully lived. That is what Jesus wants us to do. He said, "My purpose is to give . . . a rich and satisfying life" (John 10:10). And Moses would echo, "Oh, that you would choose life!" (Deuteronomy 30:19).

How we choose to view this life stage is one choice no one and nothing can take from us. Every age can be a joy—if we choose to make it so. We can, through the attitude and perspective we adopt, age well or poorly. We can be joyful or woeful, grateful or grumpy. We can complain about what we don't have, or focus on what we do have. We can squander our days, or we can savor each one.

Dear God,

As I get older, it's easy to look at what I no longer have, what I no longer can do, how I no longer look, and what I've done wrong. That's not how I want to live. Open my eyes to what I have, what I can do, what parts of me look especially good, and what I've done right.

When I think of youth, I think of verve and vitality. Give me the mindset that I can still have those qualities as I grow older. Maybe not to the same extent or in an identical way, but have them nonetheless. Let me never forget that. Even at those times when my get up and go has gotten up and gone, inspire me to retain a dynamic and eager attitude and a positive perspective. Steer my thoughts to the richness my life has gained through the addition of years. Help me focus on all the joys I can still experience. Help me see myself as vivacious in my own very special way. Amen.

SECRET #4

I have the power to choose how I perceive this life stage.

5

Fulfilling My Purpose Matters

Whatever you do, do it all for the glory of God.
1 Corinthians 10:31

O ur daughter showed me a video of her bulldog sitting on a sidewalk, watching the traffic and goings-on. Her dog's head moved slowly from side to side while a time-lapse blur of activity swirled around her. That's how I had felt at times, trying to figure out my purpose in this frenetic world. But after prayer and study, I have concluded God gave all of us the same purpose in life and put in us a deep need to fulfill that purpose.

Purpose has been defined as "the reason for which something exists" (Dictionary.com). We exist because of and for God. "God is love" (1 John 4:8). He has infinite love he wants to give, so he created us humans to be his children, to love and be loved by him. God's capacity for love is so great that he fashioned us to be "as numerous as the stars in the sky" (Genesis 26:4 NIV).

> The point of your life is to point to Him. Whatever you are doing, God wants to be glorified, because this whole thing is His.   FRANCIS CHAN

His desire is, and always has been, a close, intimate, forever relationship with his children. In Eden, that relationship was broken. God wants it restored. Revelation 21:3 (NIV) tells us God's unchanging purpose and heart longing: "God's dwelling place is now among the people. . . . They will be his people, and God himself will be with them and be their God." Since God's holiness and perfection cannot coexist with sinfulness, and man's sinful nature is a given, God provided a way to come to him—through the cleansing blood of his Son. Jesus confirmed, "No one can come to the Father except through me" (John 14:6).

God loves all his children, "not wanting anyone to perish" (2 Peter 3:9 NIV)—the fate of those who reject him. With vast patience, God has through the ages chosen humans to help bring all of us into eternal relationship and unity with him. As Christians, we are "a chosen people," God's very own possession, "that [we] may declare the praises of him who called [us] out of darkness into his wonderful light" (1 Peter 2:9 NIV), and lead others to him. That is his purpose and his plan. "The plans of the LORD stand firm forever, the purposes of his heart through all generations" (Psalm 33:11 NIV).

Because we are God's children, he also desires joy for us, and a "rich and satisfying life" (John 10:10), just as we desire for our children. Through Jesus and his Word, God shows us how to live in a way that will bring us those gifts. "So is my word that goes out from my mouth: It will not return to me empty, but will accomplish what I desire and achieve the purpose for which I sent it. You will go out in joy and be led forth in peace" (Isaiah 55:11–12 NIV).

Our purpose is to help accomplish God's purpose, plan, and desire for us, his children: to have a close relationship with him now, a rich and satisfying life filled with joy, bring others to know him, and live with him forever. If we follow Jesus; have a love relationship with God; live fully, gratefully, and joyfully in a way that brings him praise and honor and glory; and do what we can to lead others to Jesus, we are fulfilling our purpose. "Whatever you do or say, do it as a representative of the Lord Jesus" (Colossians 3:17). There is no way we can matter more.

Dear God,
May I never forget my purpose is to love you and live as you would
have me live, bringing you honor and praise and glory, so others will

know you too. Thank you that when I obey and follow you, you gift me with life in all its beauty, wonder, and joy, now and forever. You have planned it all so perfectly! No matter how I choose to spend my days, may my every thought, word, and action be honoring to you. Amen.

SECRET #5

**When my words and actions bring glory to God,
I have the joy of fulfilling my purpose in life.**

6

My Prayers Matter

Never stop praying. Be thankful in all circumstances,
for this is God's will for you who belong to Christ Jesus.
1 Thessalonians 5:17–18

One of the beauties of prayer is that it can be done anywhere, anytime, under any conditions. We'll never be too old to pray. Even physically limited, we can pray. And when we do, we matter greatly. "We are confident that he hears us whenever we ask for anything that pleases him" (1 John 5:14). And the more we converse with God, the closer to him we become. We're pleasing God by spending time and talking with him. We're helping others because God answers every prayer, even if not in the specific way we ask.

> A praying saint performs far more havoc among the unseen forces of darkness than we have the slightest notion of. OSWALD CHAMBERS

"My thoughts are nothing like your thoughts," says the Lord. "And my ways are far beyond anything you could imagine. For just as the heavens are higher than the earth, so my ways are higher than your ways and my thoughts higher than your thoughts." (Isaiah 55:8–9)

When should we pray? What and whom should we pray for? The answer is, anytime, anything, and anyone God puts on our hearts. Sometimes people request our prayers. Other times we pray without

21

being asked. Sometimes we pray for those we know, other times for people we've never met. We don't always learn the outcome. That doesn't matter. There's not a wrong subject, time, or place to talk with God. "In every situation, by prayer and petition, with thanksgiving, present your requests to God" (Philippians 4:6 NIV).

> **Come to me with your ears wide open.**
> **Listen, and you will find life.**   ISAIAH 55:3

Let's remember too that prayers are best as two-way communications. I treasure my morning quiet time with God. Yet recently I felt it was missing something. When I asked God what it was, I heard in my heart, "Listen." I realized then that my quiet time had become primarily a time of supplication. So I decided to spend at least ten minutes each morning just sitting and listening for God. When I did, he brought me such amazing insights that my listening time quickly expanded. Now I find myself listening far more than making requests. I talk *with* God, not just to him. Our morning time has become a beautiful gift of conversation and learning God's will. "He wakens me morning by morning, wakens my ear to listen like one being instructed" (Isaiah 50:4 NIV).

With no limit as to what and about whom we can pray, it's a sure way to matter.

Dear God,
Thank you for the gift of being able to talk with you any time, any place, about anything. Remind me to not just ask but also listen to whatever you want to bring to my heart. Thank you for the wisdom and guidance you so faithfully give. Thank you also that through the power of prayer I can help move life's mountains. In this new chapter of life, may I stay continually connected to you through prayer. Open my eyes, ears, and mind to awareness of those who need prayer. Thank you for the opportunity to help by lifting them up to you, and for the comfort of knowing that when I do, you will

answer with the right answer at the right time. What a gift that through my prayers I grow closer to you as well. Amen.

SECRET #6

My prayers are important and powerful.

7

Sharing My Faith Matters

So beginning with this same Scripture, Philip
told him the Good News about Jesus.

Acts 8:35

"I'm so confused. I don't know where to turn. What should I do?"
My friend looked at me pleadingly. After thirty years of marriage,
she was getting a divorce.

"I think you should ask God," I said. She looked at me quizzically.
My friend was lost. She was trying to go it alone. So I told her what
my relationship with God has meant to me, how I could never have
gotten through life's trials without him.

> God's plan for enlarging his kingdom is
> so simple—one person telling another
> about the Savior. Yet we're busy and full of
> excuses. Just remember, someone's eternal
> destiny is at stake. CHARLES STANLEY

What better gift can we give another than to encourage them to
seek, find, and know the Lord? If you are shy about sharing your
faith, ask yourself if your reticence might result in that person's losing
eternal life with God.

The longer we live, the more opportunities we may have to share
our faith. Tumultuous times can provide openings, for they tend to
unlock minds. What we say to others about God matters—to them
and to God. "If someone asks about your hope as a believer, always
be ready to explain it" (1 Peter 3:15).

God "does not want anyone to be destroyed" because they don't know him (2 Peter 3:9). He is relying on us to bring others to him (Matthew 28:19–20). It matters that we do our part in whatever way we are able. If we bring even one person to the Lord, heaven celebrates. "There is more joy in heaven over one lost sinner who repents and returns to God than over ninety-nine others who are righteous and haven't strayed away!" (Luke 15:7).

I'm not advocating standing on a sidewalk waving our Bible or cornering strangers to tell them the good news. I'm just suggesting we keep alert to chances to listen and share our hearts when the time is right. We will feel God's nudge when it is.

> **You are the only Bible some unbelievers will ever read.** JOHN MACARTHUR

God wants us to demonstrate our faith by our actions, not just our words. "What good is it . . . if you say you have faith but don't show it by your actions?" (James 2:14). When our lives exhibit the beauty of walking with God, we can increase God's kingdom, for (as Peter wrote to believing wives of unbelieving husbands) "godly lives will speak . . . without any words" (1 Peter 3:1). What a beautiful way to matter!

Dear God,
May I never hesitate to share my faith and your Word. Help me not to keep silent when I see that someone does not know you. Nudge me when the time is right, and give me the words to say. Remind me to share my faith not just through words but by how I live. May I never let concern over how I will be received allow others to perish eternally because they have not heard or understood the truth. Lead me to share my faith gently and openly, realizing there is no way to matter more to others and to you. Amen.

SECRET #7

I have the ability to help save someone's soul!

8

My Experience Matters

Wisdom belongs to the aged, and
understanding to the old.

Job 12:12

On one of TV's singing competitions, I've sometimes heard judges tell a younger person his or her performance lacked feeling. It's understandable, the judges add, because the contestant hasn't yet lived long enough to have experienced the emotions the song deals with. Similarly, a beginning pianist might accurately play all the notes from the written score, and the result may be pretty, but complexity, variety, proficiency, and emotion come from experience. What emanates from the piano of an accomplished pianist has a richness unobtainable in the early learning years.

> **Old age is not a disability or a disease.** REV. DR. RICHARD GENTZLER JR.

That's another beauty of growing older. We have experienced most all emotions many times over, giving our lives a profundity only maturity can bring. Age brings a depth of awareness, gratitude, empathy, and understanding that those who haven't been immersed in the ocean of life don't have. "The glory of the young is their strength, the gray hair of experience is the splendor of the old" (Proverbs 20:29). Our life experience has provided fuel for the fire of our passion, which we can apply to every area of our lives.

Let's celebrate that at our age, when we sing our life song, we can sing it with genuine feeling—because we've been there. And that is beautiful!

Dear God,

Layer upon layer you have built my life, giving me a richness and depth of character formed by having felt a wealth of emotions. Thank you that as I grow older, more and more beauty is transferred to my inner being. Thank you for my life experiences, which have enabled me to comprehend and value more deeply all the wonders of living. Help me appreciate the opulence of experience with which I have been gifted. May I sing the rest of my life song with gusto. Amen.

SECRET #8

My life experience has given me understanding and depth of character.

9

I Have the Wealth That Matters

Do not store up for yourselves treasures on earth. . . .
But store up for yourselves treasures in heaven. . . . For
where your treasure is, there your heart will be also.
Matthew 6:19–21 NIV

God has nothing against money and material wealth—unless they become a priority in our lives. The Bible tells us, "Don't love money; be satisfied with what you have" (Hebrews 13:5). While it's nice to have financial security and possessions, they are not the wealth that matters.

> **God will meet all your needs according to the riches of his glory in Christ Jesus.** PHILIPPIANS 4:19 NIV

Our real riches are our relationship with the Creator, our health, family, friends, and everyday life in God's magnificent world. Our treasure lies in the love, grace, and mercy of our God. "Oh, the depth of the riches of the wisdom and knowledge of God!" (Romans 11:33 NIV). Every one of us has boundless wealth regardless of the size of our bank account or the amount or quality of our material possessions.

> When I look at the night sky and see the work of your
> fingers—
> the moon and the stars you set in place—

what are mere mortals that you should think about
them,
human beings that you should care for them?

Psalm 8:3–4

Our wealth surrounds us in sunrises and sunsets, the seasons, clouds, rain, flowers, the caress of a breeze, the lilt of birdsong. It's in the trees, the mountains, and the rivers. It's laughter, a hug, a baby's silken skin and crooked smile, a blossom's lush perfume, a squeeze from the hand of someone we love, a smile meant just for us, the wag of a dog's tail, the crunch of an apple, the juiciness of a peach, and a million other delights within our reach. "O Lord, what a variety of things you have made! In wisdom you have made them all" (Psalm 104:24).

We need only open our eyes and hearts to our wealth. "Stop and consider the wonderful miracles of God!" (Job 37:14).

In the face of a loss, serious illness, crisis, or tragedy, we'd not hesitate a second to give up all the material wealth we own just to undo what we're having to deal with, just to return to the priceless beauty of each day we have been given.

"Oh normal day, what a treasure you are!" To that I say, Amen!

Dear God,

Thank you for the pleasure and comfort of possessions—but may they never blind me to my true treasures. I give you praise for the luxury of time to open my eyes to all you have blessed me with. Help me not to put great importance on what the world considers wealth. May I never be sucked into an obsession with earthly accumulations nor use them to measure how wealthy I am. For that assessment, I look to you, the beauty of your creation, and the relationships and love with which I am embraced each day. These are my true wealth, and I am wealthy indeed. Amen.

SECRET #9

I have immense and priceless wealth!

10

It Matters That I've GOT It Now

Do not dwell on the past. See, I am doing a new thing!
Now it springs up; do you not perceive it? I am making
a way in the wilderness and streams in the wasteland.

Isaiah 43:18–19 NIV

How much time do you spend thinking about yesterdays or tomorrows instead of zeroing in on the present? Take a few minutes right now to look around and absorb every delightful thing that surrounds you. What is happy and good in your current life? Take a deep breath. Appreciate how it feels. Now, take a few moments to think only about the past. Focus on a memory, pleasant or unpleasant. When you did that, what happened to your enjoyment of now and your awareness of current blessings?

Reminiscing can warm our hearts. It can also teach us and open our eyes to how far we've come. But if, instead of healthy looking back, we pine for lost youth or rehash past errors, we can miss today's joys. "Don't long for 'the good old days.' This is not wise" (Ecclesiastes 7:10).

Whether our past held bad, good, or both, we are meant to derive enjoyment and learn from it but not wallow in it. God has gifted us with a constantly evolving life and character.

The past is called the past for a reason.*

---

* This advice is not meant to minimize injurious past events or circumstances such as abuse or neglect. If you've experienced trauma, please talk to a trusted counselor or health care provider about appropriate steps to health and healing.

> **God will meet you where you are in order to take
> you where He wants you to go.**   TONY EVANS

I have a friend whose earlier married years were filled with anger, bitterness, and argument. "How are things now?" I asked. "Oh, they're so much better. We've both learned to accept and love each other for who we are. We're having the best years we've ever had. Oh, how I wish we'd woken up sooner. I can't stop reliving things I wish I could go back and change." "Whoa," I said. "Stop at 'We're having the best years we've ever had.' Live in the present; let go of the past."

But what if I don't like where I am or what I'm going through? God, through Moses, brought the Israelites out of captivity in Egypt and promised them a "good and spacious land, a land flowing with milk and honey" (Exodus 3:8 NIV). Yet it wasn't long before they were looking back, wanting to return to the past, even though theirs had been one of slavery and suffering. Because they bewailed their present and didn't trust God for their future, God allowed them to continue their desert wandering for forty years. That generation never obtained what they could have had they trusted God. Their descendants, not them, entered the land God had promised.

> **I have one desire now—to live a life of
> reckless abandon for the Lord, putting all my
> energy and strength into it.**   ED MCCULLY

Gratitude. Obedience. Trust. Lack of these prevented the Israelites from reaching their promised land. Dearth of them will keep us from reaching our promised land—the abundant life Jesus came to give us at every age. When we've GOT it—gratitude (G), obedience (O), and trust (T)—we've GOT our promised land.

Dear God,
I'm so thankful I have memories. Otherwise, I'd have to continually relearn from scratch. Thank you also for the pleasure of good memories. But if I allow them to, memories, bad or good, can smother

my present. Thank you for the past, its lessons and its joys. While my past has contributed to my now, may it never eclipse it. Let it remain a teacher or a warm, happy glow, but not become a burden to myself or others. Help me realize that my now is what counts. May I be Grateful, Obedient, and Trusting. Amen.

SECRET #10

Gratitude, Obedience to, and Trust in God will bring me the life he wants me to have.

11

My Roles Still Matter

*See what great love the Father has lavished
on us, that we should be called children
of God! And that is what we are!*

1 John 3:1 NIV

We'll always have roles. Some have altered, diminished, expanded, or disappeared. New ones have formed. We'll always be a parent of our children, but our responsibilities have changed. We'll always be the child of our own parents, but now we may also be their caregiver. As to our work, activities, and interests, our roles may be redefined many times.

It can be hard to know what some of our current roles should look like, especially when they are new or have evolved from comfortable and familiar roles into ones that feel awkward and unfamiliar. Thankfully, we can turn to God for clarity. "Open my eyes to see the wonderful truths in your instructions" (Psalm 119:18).

As with any of our roles before, it's easy to slide into our new ones without much thought, definition, or preparation. I did that in my early working years in a number of jobs. Most of us began that way in our role as a parent. But we need not do so now, for now we have the luxury of pondering.

> We do not live all these later years simply not to die. We live in order to make life better—both for ourselves and for others. JOAN D. CHITTISTER

It can be a helpful exercise to list the roles you've had over the years. Mark which ones have gone away, which remain, and which have changed. What are your responsibilities within each current role? By taking sufficient time to reflect, you may be surprised at how many roles you have today: spouse, parent, grandparent, sibling, in-law, relative, friend, church member, club member, volunteer, neighbor, community member, team or group member, and more.

Most essential, don't overlook or minimize your roles as God's child and Christ's disciple. "For his Spirit joins with our spirit to affirm that we are God's children" (Romans 8:16). "Your love for one another will prove to the world that you are my disciples" (John 13:35). We need to clearly define those roles, for they are the most important of our lives.

Dear God,

What are my roles now? That question has been chasing me.

Some of my roles are over. Help me let them go, lovingly and painlessly, appreciating that the end of those roles means the beginning of others. May I accept with grace that in some of the roles I still have, my function is changing. Reassure me, Lord, that though I'm not needed in the same ways as before, I am needed in other ways. And thank you for the new roles I've taken on. Lead me to determine accurately what they should entail. May I eagerly embrace and beautifully fill them.

Help me comprehend that the only roles I will have forever are my roles as your child, Father, and your follower, Jesus. Increase my understanding of those roles, and remind me that the way I live them will make all the difference in the rest of my life, in the lives mine touches, and in my eternity. May I put my role in your kingdom above all other roles, and make sure it impacts each one of the rest. Amen.

SECRET #11

My role as God's child and Jesus's disciple is the most important of all.

12

The Rest of My Lifebook Matters

"I know the plans I have for you," declares the
LORD, "plans to prosper you and not to harm
you, plans to give you hope and a future."

Jeremiah 29:11 NIV

Jesus did not say, "I have come that they may have life, and have it to the full until they reach age sixty. From there it's downhill." God did say, "Even to your old age and gray hairs I am he, I am he who will sustain you. I have made you and I will carry you" (Isaiah 46:4 NIV).

God created life to have different stages. He filled each with unique pleasures. He made "a time for everything, and a season for every activity under the heavens. . . . He has made everything beautiful in its time" (Ecclesiastes 3:1, 11 NIV).

The book of our life isn't finished. We've completed numerous chapters. Some we'd rather skip; others are a joy to reread. As we look over the manuscript of our days, we can ask God where it could have read better. He won't hold those portions against us. There are still blank pages, more to be written. Our life's book can't be edited, but its storyline can be continued or changed. It's up to us. We can more carefully fill our remaining blank pages, being more deliberate about what we say and do, about what the rest of our story will contain. We can stay alert and watch out for our "enemy the devil" who "prowls around like a roaring lion looking for someone to devour" (1 Peter 5:8 NIV).

> **Your present circumstances don't define where you can go; they merely determine where you start.** NIDO QUBEIN

To get started on the rest of our life book, it helps to practice the following:

- Accept that getting older is something new for us and that it takes time to adjust.
- Direct our efforts toward showing others they matter rather than wondering whether we matter.
- Stop caring what the world thinks. Care what God thinks.
- Remind ourselves that being at a new life stage doesn't mean we don't matter; we just matter in different ways.
- Focus on the good. Say out loud as often as we need to, "I have so much to be thankful for and so much to look forward to."
- Never forget that our true purpose in life is to bring glory to God.
- Pray, remembering that prayer is a conversation, not a wish list.
- Share our faith.
- Appreciate the richness our life experiences have given us.
- Realize how wealthy we truly are.
- Live in the present.
- Be Grateful, Obedient, and Trusting (GOT).
- Define our current roles and strive to fulfill them with excellence.
- Ask God what his plans are for us going forward and what our next steps should be—and then do them!
- Look to the future with confidence.

If we let God help us write the rest of our life story, then when the final lines are composed, our book will stand as a thing of beauty, a legacy for those who follow. It's not too late. And it matters.

Dear God,

Let me never lose sight of the fact that an enormous amount remains for me to experience, learn, accomplish, and enjoy. May I make the most of this new stage of my life. Help me look back with mercy and gratitude, and forward with excitement and anticipation. Open my eyes to all I have and to the dearness of each moment. Help me focus on the good, for there is so much. Give me the direction and the wisdom not to squander any part of my life. Guide me so my remaining chapters become the most glorious ones in my life's book. Shine the light of your truth into the questions and doubts that taunt me. Show me how I can yet add value in this world.

Help me see that I am a critical piece of a much larger puzzle in which, without me, there would be a noticeable space, a conspicuous gap. Show me how I fit into the bigger picture. Reveal to me what I can do to continue to fulfill your plan for my life. Show me how to contribute in a way that has impact for you, a way that will enlarge your kingdom and bring you glory. Amen.

SECRET #12

It's NOT too late!

13

My Aging Well Matters

Being confident of this, that he who began
a good work in you will carry it on to
completion until the day of Christ Jesus.
Philippians 1:6 NIV

The phrase "fine aged wines" led me to believe that aging improves wine. Then I read a Wikipedia article called "Aging of Wine." For fun, every time the word *wine* was used in that article, I substituted "people" words. I think this "people-ized" version is pretty accurate!

> The aging of *people* is potentially able to improve their quality. While *people* are perishable and capable of deteriorating, complex chemical reactions . . . can alter how they smell, how they look . . . and how they impact in a way that may be more pleasing to those around them. The ability of a *person* to age is influenced by many factors including their variety, vintage, cultural practices, where they come from, and their personality and character. The condition that the *person* is kept in can also influence how well they age and may require significant time and financial investment.
>
> The quality of an aged *person* varies significantly *person* by *person*, depending on the conditions under which they've lived and the condition of their body, and thus it is said that rather than good old *people*, there are good old *individuals*.

There is a widespread misconception that *people* always improve with age, or that *people* improve with extended aging, or that aging potential is an indicator of good *people*. . . . Aging changes *people*, but does not categorically improve them or worsen them. . . .

As certain *people* age, the harshness of youth gradually gives way to a more gentle impact. . . . The resulting *person* . . . will . . . come across softer, less astringent. . . .

As a *person* starts to mature, their personality will become more developed and multi-layered. . . . Eventually they will reach a point of maturity, when they are said to be at their "peak." This is the point when the *person* has the maximum amount of complexity, . . . softening of character, and has not yet started to decay [haha]. . . .*

Bottom line: Like wine, we don't necessarily become better or wiser as we age, but we certainly can. Our goal is to age well.

Aging well brings wisdom, perspective, and the joy of mellowing. Our youthful roller coaster of emotions can evolve into a merry-go-round. Our emotions may still go up and down and around and around, but we no longer have to hold on for a dizzying ride of steep rises and rapid falls. It's a blessing that age can bring a more even temperament, softening the edges of youthful erraticism. "Then we will no longer be infants, tossed back and forth by the waves" (Ephesians 4:14 NIV). Being less thrown by circumstance, more willing to let unimportant things go, are gifts age can bring if we partner with God. Aging well can also include

- Accepting humanness, both ours and others', and letting go of it as a source of frustration.

* Adapted from Wikipedia, s.v., "Aging of Wine," last modified September 26, 2003, 13:38, https://en.wikipedia.org/wiki/Aging_of_wine. Italics mine.

- Refusing to berate ourselves for falls we had while learning to walk through life.
- Forgiving, and accepting forgiveness, and moving on.
- Realizing it's not age that alienates. It's attitude and actions.
- Remaining open to new experiences, delving deeper into "old" interests, and pursuing what our time, health, and resources allow.
- Focusing on what we have, not on what we lack.
- Maintaining a curious mind, an adventurous spirit, and an appreciative heart.
- Opening our eyes to the miracles of everyday life.

> **There are only two ways to live your life. One is as though nothing is a miracle. The other is as though everything is a miracle.** ATTRIBUTED TO ALBERT EINSTEIN

We age well when we examine our character and identify and work with God to fill the gaps between who we are and whom God wants us to be. "The Lord—who is the Spirit—makes us more and more like him . . ." (2 Corinthians 3:18). It matters.

Dear God,
I realize that some people age well and that others . . . well, just age. May I be an individual who ages well. Remind me that what I choose to believe, think, do, and say will all impact how well I age. Point me to those aspects of my life over which I have control, and lead me to live them as you would have me live them. May I reap the benefits of the wisdom of years. Help me remember that age is just a number; it's what I do with my life that matters. May I indeed be like a fine aged wine—the kind others seek out, value, and enjoy! Amen.

SECRET #13

I can choose to age well.

14

Being My Best Matters

Concentrate on doing your best for God.
2 Timothy 2:15 MSG

God, through his Son and his Word, has shown us how to be our best. "Imitate God, therefore, in everything you do" (Ephesians 5:1). Yet it's easy to get caught up in the moment and forget what God has taught us. Thankfully, he knows we're a forgetful people. Perhaps that's why the word *remember* is in the Bible over one hundred fifty times. God even sent his Spirit to remind us. Mercifully, God "looks at the heart" (1 Samuel 16:7). "He made [human] hearts, so he understands everything they do" (Psalm 33:15). "Well then, should we keep on sinning so that God can show us more and more of his wonderful grace? Of course not!" (Romans 6:1–2).

> How noble and good everyone could be if,
> every evening before falling asleep, they were
> to recall . . . the events of the whole day and
> consider what has been good and bad. Then,
> without realizing it, you try to improve yourself
> at the start of each new day.   ANNE FRANK

How terrible it would be to reach the end of life and realize we'd never been our best for God, the best we *could* have been despite our imperfections. I want to stand before God some day and hear, "Well done, my good and faithful servant" (Matthew 25:21). Sometimes, I'm afraid his words will be, "I gave you chance after chance, but you blew it."

The good news is that now, with fewer distractions and competing demands, we can set our behavior and character as top priorities. We can ask ourselves and God, "What does *my* best look like?" (The self-assessment in chapter 15 can help with this.) Throughout each day we can ask ourselves, "Am I really, truly doing my very best?" That will help us recognize earlier when we're sliding, so we can reach out to God sooner. We'll never achieve perfection, but as long as we partner with God, we'll continue to make progress, knowing that when we slip, he'll set us back on the right path. "The LORD directs the steps of the godly. He delights in every detail of their lives. Though they stumble, they will never fall, for the LORD holds them by the hand" (Psalm 37:23–24).

> **You can't go back and make a new start, but you can start right now and make a brand new ending.**   JAMES R. SHERMAN

God is a God of second and third and many chances. But the more years we accumulate, the closer we get to the day when there are no more chances. Meantime, God will not give up on us. So let's not give up on ourselves. Today is a new day to do and be our best. It matters for us, for others, and for God.

Dear God,

I haven't always made the effort to be the best I can be. Thank you for your patience and for loving me no matter what. You've taught in your Word to forgive countless times, and that's what you've done for me. Thank you. But as the day I stand before you gets closer, I don't have the luxury of as many second chances. Even if I did, I don't want to need them. Though I'll never be flawless, I want to be everything I am able to be for you. That takes power beyond what I have, so I ask for that now. Each stage of my life has held joy, sorrow, challenge, trial, victory, failure, adventure, firsts, lasts, and everything in between. All have contributed to who I am now. But regardless of years, the clay of my life is not yet dry. I give it anew to you, for you are still the potter. I am still your clay. Lead me into new experiences, further adventures, fresh lessons, and fascinating opportunities. Throughout them all, help me live as you would have me live. Right this moment I place being my best for your glory at the top of my bucket list. If I do nothing else, may I, with your help, accomplish that goal. Amen.

SECRET #14

**I don't need to be perfect. I just
need to be my very best.**

15

My Self-Assessment Matters

LORD, . . . all we have accomplished is really from you.
Isaiah 26:12

A blessing of this life stage is having more time to reflect on who we've become, to appreciate our good, and to work on changing in ourselves what should be changed. "Search me, O God, and know my heart. . . . Point out anything in me that offends you, and lead me along the path of everlasting life" (Psalm 139:23–24).

Several years after our children left home and I'd completed my career, I was feeling discouraged. In the past, three children and a high-stress job had kept me jam-packed busy; now I felt unproductive. Tired of berating myself, I decided to inventory what I had accomplished. I was pleasantly surprised. My list revealed I had been used to nonstop activity for so long that I had interpreted slowing down as getting nothing done. Not so. My achievements were now just reasonably paced and sanely spaced, interspersed with relaxation and the luxury of unscheduled days.

> Lord, when I feel that what I'm doing is insignificant and unimportant, help me to remember that everything I do is significant and important in your eyes, because you love me and you put me here, and no one else can do what I'm doing in exactly the way I do it. BRENNAN MANNING

A self-assessment can be done for any time period. It can also ex-
tend to character. Sitting down with pen and a notebook, consider
what words describe the person you are. Make sure to include the
fruit of the Holy Spirit. Ask, "How loving am I? How joyful, peace
filled, patient, kind, good, gentle, faithful, self-controlled? What are
my strengths and weaknesses?"

Group your strengths into one list and your areas needing improve-
ment into another. Review both lists with God. Ask him how best to
transform each weakness into a strength.

As I've reflected, things have surfaced I wish I could redo or undo.
I'm working on releasing those to God, reminding myself that "we all
fall short of God's glorious standard" (Romans 3:23). Yet despite our
shortfalls, God sees us as righteous—"not having a righteousness of
[our] own . . . but that which is through faith in Christ" (Philippians
3:9 NIV).

Put your list of accomplishments and strengths where you'll see
them often. Then turn your need-for-improvement list into a project
list. Focus on one area at a time. Write down precise action steps, and
do them.

For example, are you overly anxious? Set aside time to focus on
God and the Bible every day. Check in with God every hour and ask
for his guidance and peace. Meditate on—spend time pondering—
what God has done in the past. "Give all your worries and cares to
God, for he cares about you" (1 Peter 5:7). Are you chronically late?
Make a point of being ten minutes early to everything, or even sched-
ule all your appointments for a half hour ahead of time. Set phone
alarm reminders.

Brainstorm ways to improve in each of your project areas. And
congratulate yourself on your progress as you move closer to being
your best for God's glory.

Dear God,
Help me see clearly who this person is that my years have formed.
Clarify my strengths, my weaknesses, and my potential while help-
ing me appreciate my achievements and my uniqueness. Don't let

me be too easy on myself nor overly critical. Show me my rough edges, but point out my dazzling facets as well. Illuminate the gaps between who I am and who you want me to be. Thank you for reminding me what I have accomplished and what I can still learn and achieve. Thank you for the good in me. Help me transform the not-so-good for your glory. I'm grateful for the time to do this. Amen.

SECRET #15

I've accomplished more, and made more progress, than I think I have.

16

My Health Matters

Dear friend, I hope all is well with you and that you are as healthy in body as you are strong in spirit.

3 John 2

The older we get, the likelier we are to have something physical to deal with. Ailments run the gamut from annoying to life threatening. Whether it's through our own or others' experiences, we become acutely aware of the importance of health. It's no fun struggling with illness or physical impairment of any kind. We may find it difficult to enjoy or feel enthusiasm for much of anything. I can only begin to imagine the challenge of serious illness, though I've walked through it with several people.

We're all at various places on the spectrum of health and physical well-being. When we were younger, we may have taken good health for granted. If we still have our health now, we can appreciate and revel in it, aware that many are not so blessed.

> Many people ruin their health and their lives by taking the poison of bitterness, resentment, and unforgiveness. JOYCE MEYER

Whatever our situation, it's our obligation to care for our bodies and health as best we can. That includes reasonable exercise, a healthy diet, minimal bad stress, sufficient sleep, and staying intellectually active. Our bodies "were made for the Lord, and the Lord cares about our bodies" (1 Corinthians 6:13). We can do what we're able, accepting and respecting our limits, not fighting them. The trick is to accurately determine what those limits are, not over- or underestimating them. We can live the Serenity Prayer, accepting what we cannot change and changing what we can, for age is giving us the wisdom to know the difference.

Our bodies will inevitably decline to some extent with advancing years. But through our actions and attitude, we can usually slow that decline. The Bible tells us, "Do not be wise in your own eyes; fear the LORD and shun evil. This will bring health to your body and nourishment to your bones" (Proverbs 3:7–8 NIV). The rewards we will reap from doing everything we can to maintain and improve our health will far outweigh the effort it takes. And we will be honoring God in the process. "Your body is the temple of the Holy Spirit. . . . So you must honor God with your body" (1 Corinthians 6:19–20).

Dear God,
Thank you for this body that houses my soul. May I respect it and take good care of it. The older I get, the more acutely aware I am of what a treasure good health is. May I always appreciate its dearness. Though not everything concerning my health is within my control, guide me to do all that is within my ability to keep myself healthy. Help me accept whatever true physical limitations I have but not restrict myself through laziness or unwarranted fear. Let me never sacrifice my health at the altar of indulgence or ease, but give me the guidance and self-discipline to care for my health as the irreplaceable gift it is. Amen.

SECRET #16

I need to accurately determine my physical limits, neither under- nor overestimating them.

17

My Exercise Matters

*I'm running hard for the finish line. I'm giving
it everything I've got. No lazy living for me!
I'm staying alert and in top condition. I'm not
going to get caught napping, telling everyone
else all about it and then missing out myself.*

1 Corinthians 9:26–27 MSG

A recent Facebook post said, "I did a push-up today! Well, actually I fell on my face and had to push myself up with both arms. I need chocolate." I thought it was funny but also kind of scary. For many, that post is fairly accurate.

At all ages, exercise is crucial for optimal health. Workouts for an eighteen-year-old and a seventy-year-old will differ, but both need exercise. Obviously, besides staying current with checkups and respecting any medical conditions we may have, we need to ensure our doctor approves of our exercise regimen. But how many people don't even have one? God didn't create us to be sedentary. We're to walk with the Spirit, not sit with the Spirit! Unless we're physically unable, we need to keep moving throughout our lives. The older we get, the more we need exercise to put the brakes on decline. We'll feel, look, think, love, and live better. It takes discipline, but it's worth it.

> No discipline is enjoyable while it is happening—it's painful! But afterward there will be a peaceful harvest of right living for those who are trained in this way. So take a new grip with your tired hands and strengthen your weak knees. (Hebrews 12:11–12)

> **If you can't fly, run; if you can't run, walk; if you can't walk, crawl; but by all means keep moving.**   MARTIN LUTHER KING JR.

If you have true physical limitations, just do what you're able. Keep moving in some fashion. If you're not used to exercise, begin small. Improve in manageable increments. Even adding one minute each day adds up. Once begun and consistently adhered to, exercise can be addicting. That's because it's so good for us. "I discipline my body like an athlete, training it to do what it should" (1 Corinthians 9:27). Age-appropriate, consistent exercise will create more vitality and, likely, improved health and longer life.

God can give us the power to put in the effort and self-discipline it takes. "This is the same mighty power that raised Christ from the dead" (Ephesians 1:19–20). Wow—that should be enough to keep us going!

Dear God,
You have given me this one body to last my lifetime. Thank you for it, in whatever shape it's in. It's alive and functioning, and for that I'm grateful. May I do everything I can to keep it in good working order. Please help me, through whatever hard work it takes, to make my body even stronger and healthier. May I never use "I'm too old" as a shield to hide laziness or lack of self-discipline. Help me appreciate why consistent exercise is vital for me. Establish in me the self-discipline to give my body the exercise it needs, so I can stay fit and healthy while I'm here on earth. If my resolve becomes flabby, push me to get up and get going, knowing that the benefits will far outweigh any temporary inconvenience or discomfort. Amen.

SECRET #17

I need to keep moving.

18

What I Eat Matters

*"Please test us for ten days on a diet of vegetables
and water," Daniel said. "At the end of the ten days,
see how we look compared to the other young men
who are eating the king's food."... At the end of
the ten days, Daniel and his three friends looked
healthier and better nourished than the young men
who had been eating the food assigned by the king.*
Daniel 1:12–13, 15

There was a time when, blessed by a high metabolism, I ate as many treats as I wanted and did not gain weight. But what was I doing to my body? Low blood sugar swings left me clammy and shaking. I was somewhat wiser when I became a mother, but I was still not a nutritional whiz. Now I've studied and learned more about healthy eating. Fresh, nutritious food has become a lifestyle for me. I've learned that healthy, unprocessed foods are delicious and satisfying. The more you eat them, the more you want them, and the less sweets appeal.

> Eat right.
> Respect your body.
> Dance forever.
> ELIZA GAYNOR MINDEN

But healthy eating involves vastly more than cutting down on sweets. Our bodies have nutritional needs in order to function at their best. If you don't know much about healthy eating, learning about it is a wise investment of your time. Resources abound, both in books and on-line. Discover the importance of macronutrients and micronutrients, the dangers of processed foods, which foods to avoid, and which will maximize your health. Be deliberate and educated about what you put into your mouth. Read food labels. Ask your doctor if you need supplements. Increasing your knowledge can offer a huge return.

Healthy eating, along with regular exercise, gives your body the respect it deserves. It makes you feel better so you can do and enjoy more. It's not too late to begin. And it matters.

Dear God,

It's easy to turn to food that tastes good but isn't good for me in the long run. Give me the fortitude to say no to those foods and drinks that will give me momentary pleasure but long-term problems. Remind me that what I eat matters for my health and my quality and length of life. Thank you for the abundance of food that's not only delectable but good for me. Enlighten me on the importance of eating well. Steer me toward fresh, healthy foods and away from processed, sugary, and nutritionally empty food. When I indulge in occasional treats, let me remember that their infrequency is what makes them special. Help me adhere faithfully to a healthy lifestyle, even when I'm tempted to give up or revert to easier habits. Remind me that I only get one body and one life, Lord, and that the two impact each other. May I make both the best they can be. Amen.

SECRET #18

What I eat greatly impacts my life.

19

What I Make of Mealtimes Matters

So go ahead. Eat your food with joy, and drink your
wine with a happy heart, for God approves of this!
Ecclesiastes 9:7

One evening, Jesus's disciples encouraged him to send away a huge, hungry crowd so they could go buy food in the local villages. "Jesus replied, 'They do not need to go away. You give them something to eat'" (Matthew 14:16 NIV). I can identify with the disciples' bewilderment. In my married years, I've been responsible for preparing over fifty thousand meals. So I'm sure I've frequently had the same blank stare they must have had, not only because I had so many mouths to feed with so little food but also because preparing more meals sometimes feels overwhelming.

One empty-nester advantage is no longer having to please as many different taste buds. We can stick to what my husband and I like. Yet it's easy to decide that "back to dinner for two" or "now that it's only me" means our role as meal planners, cooks, and servers no longer matters. It does!

> I decided there is nothing better than to enjoy food and drink and to find satisfaction in work. Then I realized that these pleasures are from the hand of God. ECCLESIASTES 2:24

My husband wouldn't cook a meal if it jumped on the stove. He's also not a nutrition expert. So my cooking still matters, and if you can identify, then so does yours. (If you're lucky enough to have a spouse who cooks, appreciate that gift!) If you live alone, you can have the fun of catering to your personal tastes.

Now, instead of wildly throwing items into a grocery cart in order to get home in time to feed a demanding brood, we can stroll and peruse the market aisles. We can experiment. I recently made it a point, each time I bought groceries, to purchase something I'd never tried. Some things I liked; some I didn't. All were fun to sample.

Then there's trying to figure out what to serve. I run out of ideas and get in a rut. One idea is to make just one new recipe every week or two. If you don't enjoy poring over cookbooks, hunting recipes online provides endless ideas and can be targeted to specific ingredients.

Meals are a time when we can relax with our spouse or friends. We needn't make them a big production. Still, we can take pleasure in, and please others with, food presentation—maybe some extravagance we once had no time for, or perhaps a fresh garnish that says, "I care." And what good are our best dishes when they're just sitting on a shelf? Let's use and enjoy them, even if we're by ourselves. Colors, serving dishes, and food arrangement can add enjoyment. Little things add up and can make a mealtime special.

We'd all enjoy the luxury of just sitting down each day and having delicious meals presented to us. (I guess that's called being on a cruise.) So when we're not in the mood to cook, we can eat out, simple or fancy, and relax, talk, laugh, or if we're alone, just enjoy the surroundings.

Mealtimes still matter. And we matter because we can make them something to look forward to.

Dear God,
In a world where many are starving, you have bountifully provided us with food. I sometimes look on meal planning and preparation as a burden instead of a blessing. Forgive me for those times when I've turned this privilege into a pain. Open my eyes to the importance of my role in choosing, preparing, and serving good food. Remind me that, through my efforts, meals not only can be nourishing but can

enhance our lives, provide enjoyment, and keep us connected with family and friends. Help me appreciate your gift of plenty, which takes eating beyond a mere necessity to an experience and a delight. Let me revel in the profusion of choices you've given. Inspire me to fulfill my part in providing daily bread, and to live with gratitude that I have more than enough. Thank you, God, for food. For choices. For abundance. And for the honor of being the one who can make it all come together. Amen.

SECRET #19

A little effort goes a long way.

20

How I Look Matters . . . to an Extent

How beautiful you are, my darling! Oh, how beautiful!
Song of Solomon 4:1 NIV

What about our appearance? I've struggled with that question as I've watched my wrinkles give birth.

When we request a senior price and no one argues (or worse, don't request it and are offered it); when we maintain a groundless hope that anti-wrinkle creams will make us look like smooth-skinned models . . . we would do well to head back to God's Word.

> Don't be concerned about the outward beauty. . . .
> You should clothe yourselves instead with the beauty
> that comes from within, the unfading beauty of a
> gentle and quiet spirit, which is so precious to God.
> (1 Peter 3:3–4)

The Bible says to "look beneath the surface so you can judge correctly" (John 7:24). But that does not translate to "Don't care how you look." Looking our best helps us act our best. Even when no one sees us, when we know we look less than our best externally, our internal self may deflate a notch; our insecurities may surface and reflect in our actions.

> When you do something noble and beautiful and
> nobody notices, do not be sad. For the sun every
> morning is a beautiful spectacle, and yet most of
> the audience still sleeps. ATTRIBUTED TO JOHN LENNON

Our goal is not to reverse the clock. It's to be the most amazing version of our age we can, through reasonable effort, be. That doesn't mean gobs of makeup, over-the-top trendy clothes, or limping around from exercise overload. It means simply making the effort to look our best, which tells others that we matter, and that they matter to us.

At an exhibition of works by Dutch master painters, I reflected how, for untold hours, they had meticulously applied layer after layer of paint to their canvases, creating masterpieces. Like those masters, the years have applied their strokes to our bodies and faces to create the works of art we are. No boring blank canvases. Telling ourselves, "It doesn't matter anymore," is not honoring to God. "We are God's masterpiece" (Ephesians 2:10).

Dear God,

Encourage me to accept with grace that I'm not always going to look young. Thank you for the gift of the years reflected in my face and in my body. I care how I look, and I think that's good, but teach me to pay more attention to my character than to my physical appearance. Help me assimilate and radiate the truth that genuine beauty comes from within. I do want to be my best physically, but rescue me from fixating on my outer appearance. Show me how to place sufficient importance on it—not too much, not too little, but just the right balance. Encourage me to embrace the age I am, and to be the best version of it I can be. Remind me also that who I am inside is reflected in my face, that a stern and hard heart creates a stern and hard face, and a joyful heart devoted to you creates radiance at any age. Help me remember that age is a worldly concept. So often we search vainly for eternal youth when all we need is to turn to you. Let any obsession I have with my appearance become a reminder that I'm looking too much to this world and not enough to you. When I feel old, may it prompt me to look to you and be reminded that I am your masterpiece. Amen.

SECRET #20

My appearance impacts my actions.

21

My Hands Matter

In her hands she holds the distaff and grasps the
spindle with her fingers. She opens her arms to
the poor and extends her hands to the needy.

Proverbs 31:19–20 NIV

On a cruise, I was in the photo gallery looking at a picture of our dinner table group. I asked the saleswoman how old she thought one of the women in it was. She studied her face. "Forty-five?" she guessed. "Almost eighty," I said. The saleswoman looked closer. "Oh, yes," she said. "I see it now. Look at her hands."

Hands. We can sometimes hide the age in our faces but not in our hands. Yet, let's not be unfair to hands, for they carry the story of our lives.

My hands, newborn, clung to my mother as I met the world. They explored, warned me of things too hot, cold, sharp, or rough. They brought food to my mouth. They grasped a pencil as I learned to write, were held high in response to teachers' questions. They clapped in delight. They were engulfed by my parents' hands as we walked.

My hands entwined with others' hands as I tried on love. They joined with the strength of my husband's hands as we pledged our lives to each other. They cleaned and washed, picked up, put down, carried, wrote, typed, drew, played instruments, and threw balls. They waved joyous hellos and difficult goodbyes. They steered cars and lifted groceries. They held, hugged, and caressed. My hands have dropped, retrieved, handled, chopped, directed, created, pinched, counted, squeezed, crafted, sorted, clenched, lifted, let go, stroked, stirred, dug, turned on and off, paid, pried, fetched, buttoned, glued, tied, torn, and so much more.

My hands touched our babies' silken skin, soothing and reassuring each child. They held our children, encompassed their hands, pushed them in strollers and on swings, guided their bikes as they learned to ride, turned pages on bedtime stories, and gently brushed their foreheads as I kissed them goodnight.

> **God has given us two hands—one to receive with and the other to give with.**   BILLY GRAHAM

My hands tickled tummies, administered assistance, applied Band-Aids over boo-boos, and felt fevers. They applauded accomplishments. They pointed, punished, and prompted. They wiped tears from my children's eyes and from my own, both in sorrow and in joy.

My fingers entwined with those of my son as I danced with him the day he became a husband. My hands held those of my daughters as I kissed them on their wedding days. They cuddled my newborn grandchildren. They wrapped around tender young fingers as those grandchildren grew and we walked together on their journey into life.

My hands have held my face through sobs, been raised in praise to God, and clasped in fervent prayer. They have reached out to connect me with my family, my friends, the world, and my Lord.

Our hands show our age because they have been our point of contact through all our years. We can look at them and see the totality of our life, held in God's hands and reflected in our own. "I will praise you as long as I live, lifting up my hands to you in prayer" (Psalm 63:4).

What is the story your hands manifest? What memories do they carry? Are you giving them the appreciation they deserve?

Dear God,
When I look at my hands and think, "They look so old," remind me
what they've done for me. My hands have reached out and held the
very life of life. They have touched what has held the most meaning

for me on this earth. They have sought you in prayer. My hands mirror memories. May I respect my hands and how they look, for they reflect a life that has been, and is being, fully lived. They reveal all that you, in your grace, have allowed me to experience. I thank you for my hands, Lord, and for all the moments they attest to. May I never be embarrassed by their appearance, for they reflect my abundant life. Thank you for the amazing gifts they are, for all they have done, and for all they still can do. Thank you for the joy of feeling my hand in the hand of ones I love. And most importantly, thank you that they hold your own hands, now and forever. Amen.

SECRET #21

**I should appreciate my hands, for
they reflect the story of my life.**

22

My Laughter Matters

We were filled with laughter, and we sang for joy.
Psalm 126:2

My daughter received in the mail a dress she ordered online. Let's just say it did not look like the photos. And it was several sizes too large. FaceTiming me, she pulled it out at the side and asked, "Want to join me in here? There's plenty of room." She wrapped it around her head, and I roared with laughter. It felt so good.

In the midst of our dailiness, let's not forget to smile, lighten up, laugh out loud, and have fun. After all, "the cheerful heart has a continual feast" (Proverbs 15:15 NIV). Laughter is a universal language. It's timeless. It's healing. "A cheerful heart is good medicine" (17:22). We can be the one who offers it.

Abraham Lincoln observed, "In the end, it's not the years in your life that count. It's the life in your years." We can put more life into every year by loosening up and keeping a playful mindset.

My husband and I are longtime friends with a couple who always make us laugh. They have a way of relating their experiences that turns ordinary into hilarious. They have no problem making fun of themselves. It feels good to be with them. They have taught us that no matter our age, our issues, or the messes we get into, we can turn many of life's downers into laughter by looking for the humor in them.

No one enjoys a negative person, full of tales of woe, who habitually points out the downside rather than the upside. We matter when we illuminate lives with spontaneity and laughter.

In a world of somber, preoccupied, and angry faces, how wonderful when someone smiles! Be the one who does. Even if your smile is not returned, it feels good—and it matters. You may be the first to have smiled at that person in a long time. It may impact them even if they don't acknowledge it.

> **There is nothing in the world so irresistibly contagious as laughter and good humor.** *A CHRISTMAS CAROL,* CHARLES DICKENS

Instead of fretting, which "leads only to evil" (Psalm 37:8 NIV), look for the humor in circumstances. And don't hesitate to laugh at yourself!

As Christians, we have every reason to be "filled with an inexpressible and glorious joy, for [we] are receiving the end result of [our] faith, the salvation of [our] souls" (1 Peter 1:8–9 NIV). Let's notify our faces!

> **If you're not using your smile, you're like a person with a million dollars in the bank and no checkbook.** LES GIBLIN

God "richly gives us all we need for our enjoyment" (1 Timothy 6:17). Think of the gifts he has given you, gifts of every kind. How would you feel if you gave incredible gifts to your children, but they walked around with sullen faces? Now, what if they laughed with joy?

We are made in God's image. Our laughter is our joy bubbling to the surface and refreshing others as it does. That can only make God smile, for he wants us to be filled with his joy (John 17:13).

I don't know how God feels about many of today's acronyms, but there's one he likely approves of: LOL! It stands for "laugh out loud" or "lots of laughs." LOL and we'll be enriching lives—ours and others'—and pleasing God.

Dear God,
You have given me the gift of laughter. May I enjoy and share that gift every day. Remind me what a beautiful difference I can make

through joy, smiles, and laughter. Help me remember that no one is impressed when I act oppressed, but when my joy is expressed, others are blessed!

Help me look for and discover the humor in situations. May I be a light to others and greet them with a smile. May I never be afraid to laugh when laughter is appropriate, and never hesitate to laugh at myself. Let me never take myself too seriously. May the joy you've put in my heart overflow into smiles and laughter. Amen.

SECRET #22

My smiles and laughter can make the day for me and for others.

23

How I Spend My Time Matters

Make the most of every opportunity. . . .
Don't act thoughtlessly, but understand
what the Lord wants you to do.

Ephesians 5:16–17

In my living room is a large hourglass. It reminds me how quickly time moves on, that at some point my time on earth will run out, and that I should never squander my time. None of us know when the hourglass of our life will run out, but we have reached a time when our awareness that it *will* run out sinks in.

Time is easy to take for granted. Typically, as with so many things, it's only when we fear losing it that we appreciate it fully. Age helps us appreciate time. "Teach us to realize the brevity of life, so that we may grow in wisdom" (Psalm 90:12).

It's hard to define time. To take a unique perspective, try for a moment to look at time as the ability to choose and do what we want, when we want. When younger, we had little of that luxury. At some point, physical limitations may steal it from us. But right now we likely have more of that extravagance than ever. At our age (subject to reasonable financial and physical constraints), we can indeed do what we want, when we want. Isn't that ability what we've always wanted?

> We do not know what to do, but our eyes
> are on you. 2 CHRONICLES 20:12 NIV

But how do we determine how best to spend our time? Think of how we choose books from a library. We may gravitate to a certain area, like fiction, mysteries, or history. We'll pull out titles that catch our eye and read the back cover or random passages. We pick a few books, and when we get home, we read each one for as long as it keeps our interest. Some hold our attention briefly but not enough to finish. Some we devour and want more of.

Our interests and hobbies can follow a similar path. God will guide us, for he has promised, "I will instruct you and teach you in the way you should go; I will counsel you with my loving eye on you" (Psalm 32:8 NIV).

Try listing everything you might want to do, learn more about, or be involved in. Recall what you've ever enjoyed or wished you had time for. No idea is too crazy to consider. Which items on your list most attract your attention? Brainstorm ways to try them out. Once you've given them a shot, you'll know if you want to continue with any of them or move on. If you have an impulse to do something, jump in. Does travel intrigue you? Buy those tickets, or hop in your car and explore. Visit old friends. Go see Aunt Matilda. She may be a lot more fun than you remember (or maybe not).

> **Use what talents you possess. The woods would be very silent if no birds sang but those that sang best.** *THE TWO VOCATIONS,* ELIZABETH CHARLES

Sometimes we know right away what we'd like to do. Then again, we may be so used to supporting others' interests that we've lost touch with our own. Regardless, explore. And don't worry about "excelling"—that's not the point. What matters is honoring the time God has given you to discover and pursue your unique combination of interests. Do that and you'll likely have too much fun to even think about whether you matter.

Dear God,
Each day I'm more aware of how precious every moment is. Please don't let me allow the blessing of free time to turn into aimless floundering, a

waste of priceless days. Guide me to live life fully, gracefully, graciously, and gratefully, savoring every morsel of joy, so that when I breathe my last, I will have no regrets. May I view this new life chapter as a glorious adventure, one to travel gleefully with you, exploring and experiencing the wonders and opportunities you offer. What a gift to be able to choose how to spend each day! And what an enormous library of possibilities you have given me. Whatever my choices are, I want them to please you. I ask that you direct my path so it leads me where you want me to go. Thank you for time. May I treat it as the treasure it is. Amen.

SECRET #23

Treat time as the gift it is.

24

Time Wasters Matter

Why, you do not even know what will happen
tomorrow. What is your life? You are a mist that
appears for a little while and then vanishes.

James 4:14 NIV

This Scripture from James is not comforting, but we'd do well to heed it. Instead of bringing us down, it can remind us to treat every moment as precious.

The other day my husband and I got into an argument. I don't even remember what we were bickering about. I just recall it was no fun. In the midst of our squabble, it hit me: "I don't know how much time I have left on this earth. Is this the way I want to spend it?" At that point I stopped quarreling. Our dispute, whatever it was about, ceased, and we enjoyed rather than destroyed our evening together.

The older we get, the less sand the top of our hourglass contains. Why waste any of it with unpleasantness? Losing our temper, quarreling, holding a grudge, letting little annoyances get to us . . . all are lousy ways to spend our time. "The wisdom from above is first of all pure. It is also peace loving, gentle at all times, and willing to yield to others" (James 3:17). Life brings enough challenges without our aggravating them by playing the victim, placing blame, or giving vent to foul emotions. We're old enough now to know the wisdom of "Let it go."

> **Do away with the yoke of oppression, with the pointing finger and malicious talk.** ISAIAH 58:9 NIV

Here's a list of some other time wasters. I'm certain you can add to it. If you find yourself sliding into any of them, it's time to reread

James 4:14, then call on the Holy Spirit for the self-control to change course and treat every minute as the priceless and limited resource it is.

Time Wasters

Negativity

Jealousy

Taking ourselves too seriously

Interpreting everything personally

Not giving others the benefit of the doubt

Complaints

Focusing on what's wrong instead of what's right

Rehashing past issues

Unforgiveness

Impatience

Irritability

Loss of self-control

Unkindness

Resentment

Name calling

Gossip

Criticism

Pity parties

Envy

Defensiveness

Harshness

Refusing to just "let it go"

"Our days on earth are like grass; like wildflowers, we bloom and die. The wind blows, and we are gone—as though we had never been here" (Psalm 103:15–16). These are not words we want to hear. But when we find ourselves behaving in a way that invites a good kick in the pants, reading that verse can be a needed wake-up call, for "no one knows when their hour will come" (Ecclesiastes 9:12 NIV).

Dear God,
Sometimes I forget I won't always be on this earth. I act in a way that fails to respect that my time here is limited. But I want to live as joyfully and fully as possible, and to do this, I can't allow negative emotions to gain the upper hand. When I feel them rising and am about to act in a way I'll later regret, stop me, please. Open my eyes to what a waste of time it is to give in to damaging and unconstructive behavior. Remind me that my words and actions matter. Whenever I begin to eat up my earthly time with time wasters, redirect my thoughts and behavior to revere and not waste whatever time I've been given. Amen.

SECRET #24

Let it go.

25

"Wisely" Matters

Be very careful, then, how you live—
not as unwise but as wise.

Ephesians 5:15 NIV

We don't have to pursue mighty things to live wisely. Yet have you ever gotten to the end of a day and couldn't even remember what you did? I have. When our days are ours to fill, it's easy to just let them slip by, for twenty-four hours each day is a lot of time to use wisely.

What is your "wisely"? For me, wisely includes balance. Balance doesn't need to mean equal, but for me, it's good to have a mix. In a normal day, in addition to chores and quiet time, I'd like to include writing, an interest or hobby, a project, exercise, reading, and organization. Yet often my mind goes blank on specifically what to do in those areas. So I've brainstormed everything I have any interest in, from learning wildflower names to cleaning out my closet, then grouped my ideas into categories—projects, organization, and so on. I try to keep my list current, crossing off what I've done or what no longer interests me and adding new possibilities.

Sometimes, trying to fit it all in seems overwhelming. To bring perspective, I list by category what I want and need to do that day. Then I set a generous time allotment for each item. Without fail, when I add up the estimated hours, I'm still left with a significant amount of free time. Here's an example:

Get dressed: ¼ hour
Quiet time with God: 2 hours

Writing: 2 hours

Exercise: 1 hour

Read: 1 hour

Work on a project: 1 hour

Pursue an interest: 1 hour

Organization: 1 hour

Meals and meal preparation: 2 hours

Get ready for bed: ¾ hour

Sleep: 8 hours

Those activities comprise twenty hours. I still have four hours unaccounted for! This exercise can be a real eye-opener.

> **The moment flickers like the flicker of [a] lighted match. What will you do with your moment?** BILLY GRAHAM

Our mindset is important too. If we choose to sit outside and just think and look around, not because we're bored but because it brings us joy, wonderful. If there's a TV show we want to watch, great. But if we channel surf to fill time, hoping to find something we like, it's better to turn off the TV.

To use time wisely, remember the acronym PLAD:

Pray. Ask God how best to use your time.

List everything you have any interest in doing. Sort it into categories for easier reference.

Appreciate how many hours you have in a day. List what you need and want to accomplish, assign a generous time allotment for each, add up the hours, and then see how many are left.

Determine manageable steps. Not "organize the house" but "clean out one drawer in the kitchen."

Also, remember that **Relax** is a perfectly acceptable category as long as it's not overdone.

Dear God,

You've given me a priceless commodity—twenty-four hours every day to spend as I choose. There's so much to do, see, learn, and become involved in. Open my eyes and heart to the myriad of possibilities. Guide me as I explore this wonderland of potential, a luxury I didn't have in earlier years. It's like a lavish banquet; help me savor every bite. Lead me to use my time wisely and to always include special time with you. Help me recognize the difference between healthy relaxation and wasting time. May I never squander my days or drift with meaningless fillers. Lead me to what has purpose, meaning, and value, reminding me that moments and hours combine to comprise my life. My contribution need not be huge in the scheme of things; where I can brighten someone's day, lighten a burden, or evoke a smile, lead me to that opportunity to make a difference. You have given me a generous turn at living in this world of infinite variety, which you, in your boundless creativity, have designed. Show me where to go from here and how to wisely use the days with which you've blessed me. Amen.

SECRET #25

Using time wisely takes prayer and self-discipline.

26

My Passions Matter

In his grace, God has given us different
gifts for doing certain things well.

Romans 12:6

Pursuing our interests is wonderful, but unearthing our greatest passions is like finding buried treasure. What has God placed in your heart that calls your name and won't let go? What *energizes* you? What puts a smile on your face and a song in your heart?

Children and grandchildren are passions God has put in countless hearts. Those passions are vital.

> We will tell the next generation
> about the glorious deeds of the LORD,
>   about his power and his mighty wonders.
> . . . .
>   and they in turn will teach their own children.
> So each generation should set its hope anew on God,
>   not forgetting his glorious miracles
>   and obeying his commands.
>
> Psalm 78:4, 6–7

But God gives us other passions as well. Some we may have ignored, neglected, or kept hidden. Now we have time to reach inside, bring them forth, nourish them, and let them soar.

If a passion has been starved, it may need reviving. You may even have forgotten what it is. Begin by thinking about what interests you, or what has in the past. What have you enjoyed? It doesn't have to be just one thing. If you're struggling to identify your passions, ask God to refresh them in you or lead you to them. When you feel drawn to something, try it out. Does it cause you to lose track of time? If so, you're on the right track!

> **God, I have these dreams and these desires and talents, and they seem to be leading me in a particular direction. So show me where they need to shift and change to be Your dreams and Your desires.**   MICHAEL DONEHEY

God may have given us certain passions to bring us joy: "Take delight in the LORD, and he will give you your heart's desires" (Psalm 37:4). Serving others may be a way to serve him: "There are different kinds of spiritual gifts, but the same Spirit is the source of them all. . . . God works in different ways" (1 Corinthians 12:4, 6). Perhaps it's through providing companionship to someone who's lonely, or working with others toward a common goal. It could be using your voice for his glory. Maybe it's organizing, teaching, painting, writing, knitting, or developing some other expertise and sharing it. Anything is possible if God is leading. "You can make many plans, but the LORD's purpose will prevail" (Proverbs 19:21).

The apostle Paul wrote, "Whatever you do or say, do it as a representative of the Lord Jesus, giving thanks through him to God the Father" (Colossians 3:17). When we apply Paul's words to finding and following our passions, our hearts will sing. And God's heart will sing as well.

Dear God,
Please ignite the passions you have placed in my heart, and guide me in fulfilling them. Why did you choose me—me—to come to this earth? What do you want me to accomplish now that my child-rearing and career days are behind me? How should I best pursue my passions? Thank you for those passions you have given me to

enjoy. Direct my passions to accomplish the plan you have for me in this phase of my life. Amen.

SECRET #26

**There is something that ignites my soul. I
just need to uncover it and let it soar.**

27

I Matter to My Marriage

A man leaves his father and mother
and is joined to his wife.
Genesis 2:24

At my wedding, the pastor said, "Right now the future lies hidden from your eyes." There my husband-to-be and I stood, eager to embark on our unknown journey. Over forty-five years later, a large part of that hidden future is known. We've had both better and worse.

When those of us who are married said our wedding vows, we didn't know how much "better" or "worse" the future held. Time is what shows us. Our marriage may have been, and may be, grand or a grind, exhilarating or exhausting, terrific or terrible. It may be ongoing or over. Regardless, the veil that covered the yet-to-be-discovered when we said "I do" has been lifted. What do we do with that knowledge?

We've got time to reflect now, to take stock. We can rejoice in the good and learn from the bad. When we said our vows, we trusted each other, wisely or not. Our trust may have resulted in fulfillment or letdown. That's how it is with us humans: sometimes we meet or even surpass expectations, and sometimes we fall short. But God will never let us down. "Your unfailing love, O LORD, is as vast as the heavens; your faithfulness reaches beyond the clouds" (Psalm 36:5).

> **A good marriage consists of two good forgivers.** RUTH BELL GRAHAM

Even after so many married years, we have the ability to make our great marriage incredible, our good marriage great, or our not-so-good marriage the best it's been. Sure, our spouse will play a part.

But his or her behavior and attitude can be significantly influenced by us. If we are ho-hum or worse toward our spouse, our spouse will likely be that way toward us. If we think we no longer matter to our mate, perhaps our mate is getting that same message from us. If so, we need to start offering a better message. It matters. Yes, it matters a great deal—to our spouse's and our own happiness. To our children, who even as adults observe our marriage as something either to emulate or to avoid. (Even if your marriage has ended, you can set a good example of respect, remembering that your ex-spouse was once important to you and, if you have children, still is to them.)

It matters that we leave our spouse beautiful memories of us if we leave this earth first; and that, if our spouse precedes us, our own memories aren't haunted by regrets.

And, so importantly, it matters to God, who wants our marriage to last and be fulfilling.

In this new stage of life, what a gift we can offer our mate, our children, ourselves, and God by giving our marriage a high priority and, whatever its current condition, doing all we can to make it the best it can be. The next chapter offers ideas to get you started.

> **When I have learnt to love God better than my earthly dearest, I shall love my earthly dearest better than I do now.**   C. S. LEWIS

Dear God,
Years ago, my husband and I stood before you and pledged our love for and trust in each other. We didn't know then what our future held. Now, to a great extent, we do. Through it all, the better and the worse, you have loved us. May I look back with gratitude on memories made and lessons learned. May I look forward with confidence as you continue to reveal the rest of what you've planned for us. Though much still lies hidden from our eyes, I know you will be with us always. How rapidly our married years have flown. How much they have held of difficulties and of delights, of learning and

of love. Please don't let me ever take my life partner for granted nor become complacent about our love. Thank you for the history my spouse and I share. May I rejoice in the good and learn from the bad. Remind me of the treasures that still lie ahead if I always treat our love as husband and wife as the gift it is. Lead me now to do all I can to make our remaining years together joy filled. Amen.

SECRET #27

**No matter how glorious or glum my marriage is,
I can take actions now that will make it better.**

28

I Matter in My Twosomeness

*A wise woman builds her home, but a foolish
woman tears it down with her own hands.*

Proverbs 14:1

At a work reunion, I reconnected with former colleagues, many now retired. Several laughed that they married years ago "for better or for worse, but not for lunch." Though spoken as a joke, their words belied a potential unspoken truth. They may no longer enjoy being with their spouse all that much.

What happened to their excitement at being two? It may have been squelched by habits, ruts, and lack of effort. We all need some alone time. The danger lies in that need becoming our primary desire. "Let's have fun together and some space alone as well" can become "Let's avoid each other as much as possible."

A return to twosomeness is an opportunity to matter greatly. We can avoid the "I don't want them to be around me all day" mentality by reinjecting our relationship with enthusiasm and adventure.

Do *you* infuse each day with romance, delight, and enthusiasm, going out of your way to show your spouse he or she matters? It's a good time to remember God's Golden Rule: Do to your spouse what you would like your spouse to do to you (Matthew 7:12). If you make it clear you still delight in your life partner, chances are your twosomeness will glow again.

Try these connection enhancers:

- Hugs and hand holding. Creative surprise outings together. Exploring new places and attending unique events. Enjoying candle-lit dinners. Eating out (or in) without cell phones to distract.
- Being interested in what interests your spouse, and share what fascinates you. Talking *with*, not at, your mate, looking into his or her eyes when you do. Asking for your spouse's thoughts and opinions—and then listening. Treating your mate as if you've just met; getting to know your partner afresh, looking for the good and ignoring the rest.
- Laughing, smiling, snuggling, being playful, blowing your loved one a kiss. Telling him he's your knight in shining armor, or telling her she's the queen of your heart, and then acting like it's true.
- Praying together. Showing enthusiasm. Partnering to create a list of things to do, and then doing them. Writing down everything good about your spouse, and telling your spouse some of those things every day. Freely giving affection and not withholding it.

> Kiss me and kiss me again,
>   for your love is sweeter than wine
> . . . .
> You are as exciting, my darling,
>   as a mare among Pharaoh's stallions
> . . . .
> You are so handsome, my love,
>   pleasing beyond words!
> . . . .
> You are altogether beautiful, my darling,
>   beautiful in every way.
>   Song of Solomon 1:2, 9, 16; 4:7

Try saying those words, taken from the Bible, to your spouse. Your mate may look at you like you're crazy, but inside . . . how could anyone not smile?

In his poem "Rabbi ben Ezra," Robert Browning famously wrote, "Grow old along with me / The best is yet to be." It matters that we strive to make that happen and not let it become just, "Grow old with me; the rest is yet to be." If we invest the effort, our spouse will likely join us. Even if you don't get an immediate positive response, don't give up. Ask God for guidance and strength to keep at it even when you feel discouraged. "Let's not get tired of doing what is good. At just the right time we will reap a harvest of blessing if we don't give up" (Galatians 6:9).

Imagine your relationship reigniting. You can be either the spark that lights your spouse's fire or the water that douses the flame. Why settle for less than the best that your remaining years together can be? Think what an example you'll be setting for your family and friends as they see the two of you acting like you're falling in love all over again. Although it won't be acting! You matter because it's you who can make it happen.

> Look, the winter is past,
>   and the rains are over and gone.
> The flowers are springing up,
>   the season of singing birds has come,
>   and the cooing of turtledoves fills the air
> . . . .
> Rise up, my darling!
>   Come away with me, my fair one!
>   Song of Solomon 2:11–13

Dear God,
I remember the thrill of becoming a twosome. Yet as we became a family, our time and focus was often not on each other. The days stampeded. Now here we are again, back to two. Bring to our minds the joy of being a twosome again. Show me what I can do to cause the flame of our love to blaze anew. Help me remember that if I want to matter to my spouse, I need to show that my spouse still matters to me. Lift me from the ruts in my life and snap me out of

me-me-me routines. May I never forget that while we did marry for better or worse, that what I think, say, and do can make the difference between having it be better and making it worse. May I take this opportunity of time and togetherness to demonstrate, in all I say and do, that I feel blessed to be my loved one's spouse. May my thoughts, attitude, actions, and words all bring new life to the garden of love my spouse and I share. May the two of us enjoy each other fully, and may the cooing of turtledoves once again fill the air! Amen.

SECRET #28

I have the power to make my marriage sing again.

29

I Matter in My Singleness

He heals the brokenhearted and binds up their wounds.
Psalm 147:3 NIV

For years you've been one-half of two. Now you're one. Getting used to life without your spouse is difficult. It's a process. Grief is part of that process. Turn to Jesus. Cry to him, talk with him, share with him, receive his guidance, and be wrapped in his love. "Trust in him at all times. Pour out your heart to him, for God is our refuge" (Psalm 62:8).

During your married life, some things were largely or fully your spouse's responsibility. Others were yours. In other words, the two of you shared life, partnered in it. That's what you're used to. Now, without your mate, life can be lonely, confusing, frightening, even overwhelming.

> If there is something we need more than anything else during grief, it is a friend who stands with us, who doesn't leave us. Jesus is that friend. BILLY GRAHAM

While a transition to singleness will take time and effort, you can "let God transform you into a new person by changing the way you think" (Romans 12:2). This season of change can be viewed as one of personal expansion and growth. Megan Courtney, who lost her young husband to illness, puts it like this: "When I chose to accept that I wasn't Kenny's wife anymore, it was the most soul crushing, and yet liberating part of the process. Once I started making decisions with only my likes, dislikes, wants or needs, I was able to start piecing myself together again. I learned who I was now, and where I wanted my life to go."*

Widowhood, challenging though it may be, can also be a time of blessings. God has a special concern for the widowed: "Defender of widows—this is God" (Psalm 68:5). "Your widows, too, can depend on me [God] for help" (Jeremiah 49:11).

You can use your experiences to help and encourage others going through the same or similar losses. God "comforts us in all our troubles so that we can comfort others" (2 Corinthians 1:4).

Though you may feel devastated, make it a project to look for, and repeatedly remind yourself of, the good that's still in your life. It is there. Ask God to open your eyes to it. In the words of nineteenth-century hymnist Clara Scott,

> Open my eyes that I may see
>   glimpses of truth thou hast for me.
> Place in my hands the wonderful key
>   that shall unclasp and set me free.
> Silently now I wait for thee,
>   ready, my God, thy will to see.
> Open my eyes, illumine me,
> Spirit divine!

When you find your mind drawn to the negative, follow God's Word by turning your focus to what is "right . . . and worthy of praise" (Philippians 4:8).

"This is what [the LORD] requires of you: to do what is right, to love mercy, and to walk humbly with your God" (Micah 6:8). With that Scripture in mind, you now have the freedom of singleness, a green light to say yes or no to whatever you choose. Ask God to direct your paths. "Your king will lead you; the LORD himself will guide you" (2:13). Here are some ideas to get you started on your new autonomy:

---

* Megan Courtney, "Seven Motivational Quotes That Helped This Widow," Living the Second Act, October 9, 2018, https://livingthesecondact.com/2018/10/09/7-motivational-quotes-that-helped-this-widow.

- Accept your "grief bursts." They are normal and natural. Experience them, then move on.
- Say yes to invitations, and don't be shy about initiating them. Others may be trying to respect your privacy or don't know what to say, but they'd be delighted if you asked them to have coffee together.
- Is there a special interest you've neglected? Join a group or organization that shares your interest. You can look online for opportunities or create a group yourself. Don't know how? Type in "how to form an interest group."
- Step out of your comfort zone and try fresh experiences.

Look on God as your husband. "For your Maker is your husband—the Lord Almighty is his name" (Isaiah 54:5 NIV). God will love you, provide for you, comfort you, listen to you, and guide you. God can "[call] you back from your grief" (v. 6).

Dear God,
Thank you that I am never alone, that you are with me always. I know this is true, yet it's hard not to feel lonesome because I miss my spouse. I miss their presence, touch, help. I miss all the little things I too often took for granted when my mate was here. Thank you for the years we had together. Help me to remember them tenderly, and to turn to you when I'm hurting. Lead me forward, fill me with your peace and, yes, your joy. Help me use my singleness to focus on the person you want me to be and to reach my potential as an individual. When I feel overwhelmed, hold me. May I focus on all I have, and on the bouquets of possibilities you are holding out to me. Amen.

SECRET #29

Singleness can be a time of personal growth and adventure.

30

My Being
a Parent Matters

Parents are the pride of their children.
Proverbs 17:6

With the nest now empty, our role as PARENT has shrunk to that of parent. No longer are we the final decision makers, the ones in charge, an essential part of our children's every day. But though we're not the center of their lives, we remain an important part of their world as they continue the beautiful PARENT-to-parent cycle with another generation.

That our children have left should fill us with deep satisfaction. Our courtship, falling in love, marriage, childbearing, and years of family togetherness and child-raising were all intended to culminate here. Now can be our time of celebrating achievement, our critical part in God's great plan accomplished.

> **God hasn't just sent you to do his work in the life of your children; he will use the lives of your children to advance his work in you.** PAUL DAVID TRIPP

When our children were in our care, they needed us to teach them, guide them, help them, advise them. Now that they're adults, they don't *need* us for those things. But they may choose to ask us for them. Choose. That's the crucial word. And choosing is even better than needing. Now that our children are grown, when they turn to us, it's by choice, not necessity. That's a fact to cherish.

In my early transition from PARENT to parent, too often I defined my role by what *I* wanted and needed. Basically, I wanted to still be needed. I traveled through frustration, dismay, and hurt before realizing that being wanted is better than being needed. I've learned to back off and let them choose me. I think God may feel the same way. He wants to be needed. Yet more than that, he wants to be chosen.

Let's embrace the times we *are* chosen, *are* included, the times when our adult children *are* filled with questions, interest, and enthusiasm about what we're doing. Let's not worry about the rest. This has nothing to do with getting older or not mattering, only with the way life was made to be.

As I write this, sitting here in my long-empty nest, thinking of our children's adult lives unfolding, knowing they are in God's faithful care, I feel peace, profound joy, and fulfillment. I think our children do too, knowing I'm praying and that I'm watching—often at a distance, yes, but nonetheless caring for them, loving them, and here for them when they need me. I know I still matter to them . . . and it feels wonderful.

Dear God,
Our children are grown. It happened so fast. Just yesterday they were tiny and dependent upon me. Now they're independent adults. There are times when I worry whether I still matter to them. How can I be enough for them without being too much? Where and how do I fit into their lives now?

Help me understand my current role as a parent. Show me when to step in and when to step away. Give me the self-discipline to allow my children to live their lives without me hovering or interjecting. Thank you for the thrill of watching their victories and accomplishments and sharing their joys. When I see them hurting or struggling, give me the fortitude to let them experience life in all its ups and downs and to not try to protect them from its realities.

You matter to me greatly, Lord, yet often I appear to forget about you, not include you, and come to you seeking to fulfill my needs but not asking about your desires. May I remember this when I wonder whether I still matter to my children, and let it serve as my reminder to think of you and include you. I did my best to give my children a strong foundation. Help me now to stand back and permit them to build on it. Remind me that having my own life as an adult never meant I loved my parents less, nor does my children's independence mean they love me less. May I never be a burden to them by wanting more than they give. I know you understand how much better choice is than coercion. That is what you want from us. Let me be the same way with my children. Amen.

SECRET #30

Being chosen is better than being needed.

31

The Example
I Set Matters

Jotham was twenty-five years old when he became
king. . . . He did what was right in the eyes of
the LORD, just as his father Uzziah had done.
2 Chronicles 27:1–2 NIV

I identify with a post that read, "I opened my mouth and my mother came out." The older I get, the more I notice my mother in me—not only in physical appearance but also in words and behavior. While it makes me laugh, it also gives me pause, for I'm already observing myself in things my adult children say and do (though it's best not to point this out to them).

When my mother exits my mouth, I should be glad, for my mother was a gracious, loving woman. But sometimes I cringe, for like all humans, she had a few irritating things about her, and I seem to have picked up those as well. If I'm going to be like my mother, and if my children are going to be like me, I want it to be good.

> No matter how far we come, our parents are always in us. BRAD MELTZER

"Like mother, like daughter; like father, like son." Parental influence, for good or bad, is nothing new. "Amaziah son of Joash king of Judah began to reign. . . . In everything he followed the example of his father Joash" (2 Kings 14:1, 3 NIV). "[Uzziah] did what was right in the eyes of the LORD, just as his father Amaziah had done" (2 Chronicles 26:4 NIV). "Amon was twenty-two years old when he became king. . . . He did evil in the eyes of the LORD, as his father Manasseh had done" (33:21–22 NIV).

At every age, our children watch us, absorb us, and reflect us, even without realizing it or wanting to. What we do and say and the example we set matter, even when they are grown. "The godly walk with integrity; blessed are their children who follow them" (Proverbs 20:7). We can now teach them how to grow older well.

In the midst of child-rearing, we may have been too busy to give much thought to what characteristics we were passing on to our kids. It may have been years before we were either delighted or dismayed to see ourselves in their words and actions. Though our most influential years have passed, it's not too late to reinforce our good examples and correct our bad. Admitting our mistakes and changing can inspire, teach humility, and reinforce the reassuring news that until the day we die, we're *all* works in progress. Our children will appreciate that we acknowledge our humanness. What we do at every age matters. The oft-repeated maxim "Be the kind of person you want your children to be" is good advice. We can live *now* in such a way that, when our children open their mouths and we come out, it is good.

Dear God,
When I think I don't matter, open my eyes to how much of me is reflected in what my children say and do. Keep me aware that my unconscious influence on them remains to the end, and it matters. Never let me ignore the influence I have on who even my adult children are. Regardless of what's gone before, may the life I lead now have this effect: that when they open their mouths and I come out, it is good in your eyes. Amen.

SECRET #31

I am still setting an example.

32

It Matters That I Bless My Child's Marriage

Show love in everything you do.
1 Corinthians 16:14 CEV

One of my most treasured gifts from my husband is a small plaque which reads, "All Because Two People Fell in Love."

Think how many people's lives would be different or not even exist if you and your husband hadn't fallen in love. You are and can be the source of positive impact on many lives now and on countless lives to come. We fall in love, get married, and have children. Our children fall in love, get married, and have children. And on and on it goes. What a blessing to be part of this process called life.

I vividly recall holding our newborn son, our first child, and thinking how he would grow up and someday leave me for another woman. I envisioned how painful that would be. Twenty-six years later I found I'd been wrong. It wasn't painful. It was a joy! Our son fell in love with an incredible woman who is easy to love. Our two daughters also met their soulmates, men it was a joy to welcome into our family. It's a thrill to see each of our children creating a family of their own.

Our son's or daughter's marriage means he or she has found a life partner who will love and be there for our child even after we have left this earth. What a gift! We can thank God for enlarging our family, and we can enjoy our sons- and daughters-in-law as our love expands to encompass them. Our family has become a FAMILY. Even after we're gone, we will live on through them.

Whether you feel disappointment or joy over your child's choice of a marriage partner, how you react and how you treat your son- or daughter-in-law always matters. A lifetime gift to your children can be to love and support their spouses (assuming they're not abusive) and to include them sincerely and enthusiastically as part of your family. If you're critical toward a child's spouse, you may create an unbridgeable chasm, for the two are united into one.

> **Our family is a circle of strength and love, founded on faith, joined in love, kept by God.** CHRISTIANWALLS.COM

I don't understand why there are so many in-law jokes or why they are almost exclusively mother-in-law jokes. Perhaps it's a result of many mothers-in-law not respecting that their children have families of their own, and that Mom is rightly in the background now. Refusing to meddle will make it more likely we remain an important part of our married children's lives, not a subject of their jokes.

The strains a marriage experiences from the world and life are demanding enough. We don't need to add intra-family strife as well. We can matter in our married children's lives by ensuring that our relationship with them and their spouses is one less thing they need to worry about.

Dear God,
As part of your perfect plan of continuity, you have brought my child a spouse—someone to love, cherish, and grow old with; someone to live, laugh, and love with; someone to share adventures with, to care for, to bring forth life and raise a family with. What a blessing! What a joy. My child has found a soulmate, and it's my time to step aside as the most important person in my offspring's life. Help me do so with grace. Guide me to always encourage, love, and support my child, his or her spouse, and their marriage—all in the right way and right amount. Ensure that I welcome my child-in-law as another adult daughter or son. May the joy of my adult child be my

joy as well. Let me be an example of your love, Lord, and let my marriage furnish a healthy model they want to strive for. I pray that my words and actions will only add to their happiness. Amen.

SECRET #32

My child's spouse needs my love.

33

Who I Am as a Grandparent Matters

May you live to enjoy your grandchildren.

Psalm 128:6

"Y ou're going to be a grandparent!"

I'll never forget the take-my-breath-away feeling of hearing that—not only the first time but with each additional grandchild. The awe I felt was much like the wonder and thrill I experienced many years ago upon learning I was carrying each of my own children.

Being a grandparent is both a joy and a responsibility. It's an opportunity to enjoy, teach, and exemplify love, family, and the Lord. "You must be very careful not to forget the things you have seen God do for you. Keep reminding yourselves, and tell your children and grandchildren as well" (Deuteronomy 4:9 CEV). We can show our grandchildren they're a treasure, embrace them with the security of family, and open their eyes to the privilege of knowing and serving God.

Physical distance does not mean we won't matter to our grandchildren. Proximity isn't what determines closeness. When our children and grandchildren live far from us, we may even make more of an effort to see them and stay in touch. Both my maternal and paternal grandparents lived many states away. Back then air travel and even long-distance calls were seen as special events. But because they wrote to me often and ensured the times we were together were joy filled, I felt close to them and loved them dearly. They mattered to me and always will.

How much greater are today's opportunities to stay connected with our grandchildren. But it's up to us. We can live far away and still be close; we can live nearby and yet be distant. Whether near or far, "close" is ours to choose—and it's by far the better choice.

> It's funny what happens when you become a grandparent. You start to act all goofy and do things you never thought you'd do. It's terrific. MIKE KRZYZEWSKI

Without smothering, we can demonstrate we care about our grandchildren's opinions, feelings, favorite things, friends, interests, challenges, victories, and defeats. We can listen, encourage, support, and be their biggest cheerleader. We can share the parts of our lives that may be meaningful to them. We can let them know they're a joy while modeling responsibility and respect. Most importantly, we can talk with them about God. "Now that I am old and gray . . . let me proclaim your power to this new generation, your mighty miracles to all who come after me" (Psalm 71:18).

We can add value and richness to our grandchildren's lives and increase their faith. We can be grandparents they enjoy, look forward to seeing, and someday remember with love. Or we can be uninvolved and distant.

Our grandchildren are part of the continuum of life. We can show them the importance of that continuum. With God's grace, someday they will be grandparents too. With God's help, we can be grandparents they'll want to emulate. With God's love, we can matter in their lives.

Dear God,

It still amazes me that my children have children of their own. Thank you for granting me this awesome blessing of grandchildren. And, wonder of wonders, this precious new generation carries on a part of me as well. How incredible! Grandparenting is a responsibility I have eagerly taken on. Help me fulfill it with excellence. Guide me to be a grandparent who leaves the legacy of a positive imprint.

Remind me that now, without the daily pressures, demands, and stress that come with raising and providing for a family, I can focus on being an even better example of what it means to love those dearest to me and honor you. May I not intrude on my children's parenting, but offer them my support and love. May my grandchildren treasure our moments together and the memories we create. May I be constantly aware that my role as grandparent is special indeed, and that how I live it matters. Thank you for the privilege and joy of grandparenting. Lead me to be a grandparent who matters. Give me the wisdom and direction to play a significant role in my grandchildren's lives. Show me how best to stay connected to them, so that even when we're physically distant, we stay emotionally close. Amen.

SECRET #33

Grandparenting is a responsibility as well as a joy.

34

I Matter to My Parents

Each of you must show great respect
for your mother and father.
Leviticus 19:3

When we feel we don't matter anymore, we can think of our parents and how much they matter to us and always will. If we wonder whether we'll be missed someday, we need only realize how much we will miss our parents (or perhaps already miss them).

And just as our children will always matter to us, so we will always matter to our parents. God's command in Ephesians 6:2 to honor them is not age limited. If their abilities have diminished, we may need to care and provide for them as well. "Anyone who does not provide for their relatives, and especially for their own household, has denied the faith and is worse than an unbeliever" (1 Timothy 5:8 NIV).

Even if our parents are doing great, we can make a huge difference in their quality of life by showing them they still matter—something they may doubt. If we need to know we still matter, imagine how they feel. They likely crave reassurance more than we do. We can enrich their lives as they've enriched ours.

The way we treat our parents will also set an example for our children. Applying the Golden Rule a slightly different way, in everything, we should do to our parents as we would have our children do to us.

> To care for those who once cared for us is one of the highest honors. TIA WALKER

The older we get, the more we understand and appreciate our parents' love and sacrifices. No matter what our relationship with them has been in the past, we can now make their world brighter by giving them our attention and our love and never taking them for granted. Doing so today will avoid if-only-I-hads tomorrow.

Dear God,

Thank you for my parents. May I never take for granted the love and support they have given me through the years. May my every interaction with them now be honoring and loving. Help me remember that I will always matter to them and that they want to know they matter to me. Be it easy or difficult, may I care and provide for them in whatever ways they need. My parents matter greatly to me. It doesn't matter how old they are. Help me remember this when I start to wonder whether my own age makes me matter less. Amen.

SECRET #34

It's an honor to honor my parents.

35

I Matter to My Friends

A friend is always loyal.

Proverbs 17:17

Sorting through a stack of long-forgotten papers, I came across a list of friends I'd compiled more than twenty-five years ago, probably as a potential party guest list. I recognized names I hadn't thought about for years. I don't know where those persons are now or what the last quarter-century has held for them. There were also names of people who must have been a part of my life for some reason, but I don't remember them. Finally, there were a handful of names who are still my close friends. Of all the friends I've known, why have some vanished and others endured regardless of distance or time?

It's been said that people enter our life "for a reason, for a season, or for a lifetime."

Every friend we've had likely fits into one of those categories. "Many people will walk in and out of your life, but only true friends leave footprints in your heart."* It's those footprint friendships that last. Old friends can indeed be the best friends. "If one person falls, the other can reach out and help" (Ecclesiastes 4:10). Old friends are the ones with whom we've weathered life's storms, who have remained loyal and loving despite inevitable vicissitudes. We "share each other's burdens" (Galatians 6:2). We can be truly relaxed around each other. Being with such a friend is like eating comfort food. "A sweet friendship refreshes the soul" (Proverbs 27:9 MSG). Old friends are the ones we can even go long times without seeing, yet when we do, it's like we've not been apart.

* Commonly attributed to Eleanor Roosevelt.

For years, our children and careers may have taken precedence. Now our more spacious calendars can include more friend times. In this chapter of life, we have time to renew dormant friendships, nurture active ones, and even establish new ones.

> **Friendship is born at that moment when one person says to another, "You too? I thought I was the only one."** PARAPHRASE OF C. S. LEWIS

As old friends, we can unselfconsciously start yawning in the evening because our friend is yawning too. We can let go of worry about the lines on our face or our aging neck and hands because our friend has the same wrinkles. We can laugh at the same jokes, share similar stories, and understand each other's aches, pains, and life experiences. "Though good advice lies deep within the heart, a person with understanding will draw it out" (Proverbs 20:5). We can be a great source of support and reassurance to each other. It feels good to be with our old friends because we're on the same page, or at least in the same chapter, in our life books.

The longer a friendship has lasted, the greater the likelihood we and our friends will experience difficult times. Just as we cherish friends in our tough times, we matter to them in theirs. We can support, assist, encourage, and be there, blessing them through our friendship.

Friends will continue to enter our life for a reason, a season, or a lifetime. Let's never overlook the gift our friends are to us and that we can be to them.

Dear God,
Thank you for making us a people who need each other. You are a God who treasures relationships, and we are made in your image. Thank you for putting friends in my life for a specific purpose, for a particular time, or for a lifetime. Thank you for the many friends who've graced my life through the years. Thank you for the good times, the laughter, the caring, the support, and the love. Thank you most of all for my old, my longtime, and my lifetime friends. Help

me to be for them, and for all my friends, the friend I want them to be to me. May I never overlook them, neglect them, or fail to appreciate them. Keep uppermost in my mind how much my being a true and faithful friend matters, especially now. Amen.

SECRET #35

My friends need me as much as I need them.

36

My Possessions
Don't Matter

Do not store up for yourselves treasures on earth. . . .
For where your treasure is, there your heart will be also.
Matthew 6:19, 21 NIV

My mother was a saver. I think it was because she loved so deeply and had such a zeal for life. She didn't want to let go of anything that held precious memories or potential. My parents' recreation room morphed into a storage space so jam-packed with stuff that it was unusable. How I wish she had sorted and simplified, decided between the jewels and the junk. This would have helped both her and those she left behind. For when she lived, accumulation became a source of distress, a constant cloud over her head. And when she passed on, we were left to deal with her ninety-four years of possessions. It was overwhelming, so much so that, sorting through her stuff, I probably threw out the meaningful along with the meaningless. I picked a few things that spoke the most to me of her, then said goodbye to the rest. It was difficult. Sometimes it still haunts me.

I don't want to do that to my children. As Lisa J. Shultz says in her book *Lighter Living*, "Losing the buffer zone of my parents meant I was next. I had a chance to craft a lighter finale for my future senior years. I didn't want the final chapters of my life to be about stuff, and I didn't want to abandon the responsibility of dealing with it myself."*

* Lisa J. Shultz, *Lighter Living: Declutter. Organize. Simplify.* (Breckenridge, CO: High Country Publications, 2019), introduction.

My mother meant well. She never intended to make it hard. She felt her treasures would be ours as well. They might have been, had she pared them down. I think she would have been happier too, freer to enjoy what meant the most. But after my mother was gone, it wasn't her stuff I wanted. It was her. It wasn't her belongings I cherished; it was her love, her character, her essence, that I would hold forever in my heart. It was who she was, not what she had accumulated, that mattered. That is how it will be with us.

> **It is not how much we have but how much we enjoy that makes happiness.** CHARLES SPURGEON

I've learned not to hold on to things just for the sake of holding on. The momentary sting of tossing is quickly forgotten. So don't worry about saving things for posterity. Those you leave behind likely won't even want what you let go of, and you'll get greater enjoyment from what you keep.

When deciding whether to keep, give away, or discard, I ask myself one or more of these questions:

- Why do I want this or think I need it?
- Is this essential or important to my life? If so, how?
- When will I use it or enjoy it?
- Will I miss it?
- Have I already gotten all my enjoyment out of it?
- Is it taking more out of me than it's giving me? (To me, this is the most important question.)

There's nothing wrong with owning and taking pleasure in things. There *is* something wrong with merely owning but not using or enjoying things. When things engulf, obscure, or interfere with what truly matters, it's time to let them go. "Those who cling to worthless idols turn away from God's love for them" (Jonah 2:8 NIV).

Let's focus on ensuring that what we leave behind are beautiful memories. As for our stuff, we can see it for what it is—just stuff.

Dear God,
You've allowed me lots of toys in the playground of life. Some I still enjoy; others I've outgrown. Some I often even forget I have. Thank you for the fun of owning stuff and of having tangibles that bring back pleasant memories. But when I overvalue a possession or keep it for no good reason, please tell me it's time to let it go. Help me get rid of things that no longer give pleasure or have meaning. May I never force my life upon the lives of my children by expecting them to want my things. Let me never keep possessions hoping or antici-pating they will mean as much to others as they do to me. Help me focus on who I am as a person instead of what I own. May I enjoy everything I've been blessed with but keep my priorities where they should be—with you, with those I love and care about, and with the intangibles that do count. Amen.

SECRET #36

It's who I am, not what I've accumulated, that matters.

37

My Photographs and Memorabilia Don't Matter as Much as I Think They Do

*However many years anyone may
live, let them enjoy them all.*

Ecclesiastes 11:8 NIV

When I was young, picture taking was a luxury in our home. Because film and developing were considered a splurge, photographs were limited to special occasions like birthdays and graduations. People now take more pictures in one day than my family took in twenty years. Photography has become a worldwide mania.

It's easy to get caught up in this obsession. I've taken almost a thousand snapshots on just one vacation. I've thoroughly chronicled highlights as well as more mundane moments of each of our children's lives. Visits with our grandchildren have birthed many photos.

Recently, though, I've asked, What for? Sure, it's fun to reminisce occasionally, and sharing current photos keeps friends and family close. But there's no way I'll ever review all my photographs and videos. Somewhere between the paucity of my childhood memorializing and a stream of moment-by-moment visual records, there's got to be a satisfying middle ground.

The sheer volume of photos embedded in my phone and computer and crammed into boxes instills guilt in me. When am I going to get them all organized? Why did I take so many if I'm not going to look at them? Do I owe it to my family to sit down and at least distill the best for them to enjoy?

I've likely missed fully experiencing many moments because I was watching them through a camera lens or fretting over getting the perfect shot instead of absorbing the present. Now I'm saying, "Forget the photos. Enjoy the moment." There are more experiences ahead to enjoy.

> The best and most beautiful things in the world cannot be seen nor even touched, but just felt in the heart. HELEN KELLER

I took oodles of videos and photos of our kids growing up for them to enjoy as adults. I had an eye-opener when our son's first child turned one. Eagerly I unearthed the video of our son's first birthday, certain he'd be enthralled. But my pointing and excited comments ended when I saw he'd fallen asleep on the couch. Lesson learned: our kids might not be all that interested in looking back.

With that in mind, I sorted through mounds of school papers generated by our kids. Having tons had weighed on me. Keeping just one box of each child's best academic mementos is a relief. My next goal is to select one or two items per year from each box and put them in a scrapbook. Even then, chances are the book will garner only a glance and then collect dust.

I don't mean to sound negative. I'm just trying to be realistic. With photos and memorabilia, as with much in life, less is more. One photo or work of art is all that's needed to share, or to spark a memory. I rarely take the time to peruse old photos and memorabilia. Why would I expect others to? And when I do reminisce, I only enjoy it in small doses. Then it's time to move back into the present where I belong.

Do what you feel good about and enjoy, but don't be disappointed if others don't share your enthusiasm for whatever you keep or produce. It's good to reasonably document our lives. It's even better to simply enjoy them.

Dear God,

Thank you for the technology that makes it so easy to preserve memories, but help me to not let it take precedence over fully experiencing the present. As to all the documentation I've kept of the past, help me wisely determine what to keep and what to throw away. Don't let it become a burden to me or others instead of the delight it was meant to be. Show me how to distinguish between what will bring joy and what is excess. Free me to live each moment completely and not worry so much about recording it for the future. May I be an example of how to appreciate the past but not become obsessed by it. Thank you for every new adventure. Guide me to live in the now of my life. May I never be so focused on memorializing and remembering that I miss out on the present. Amen.

SECRET #37

Less is more.

38

Holidays and Other Chores: How I Handle Them Matters

So they began to celebrate.
Luke 15:24 NIV

I was ecstatic our adult children would be home for the holidays. But as I began a list of preparations, my exuberance was tempered by mild dread at the thought of lugging boxes of decorations upstairs and decorating our house.

For years I delighted in acquiring those decorations. Bedecking our home was a happy time of togetherness. But after our children left home, I began to doubt that decorating and post-Christmas dismantling were worth the effort. I was having the same mental battle with birthdays and other holidays. I no longer looked forward to searching for, unwrapping, briefly displaying, and then rewrapping and re-storing ceramic Easter bunnies and Pilgrim figurines, or to blowing up balloons and hanging streamers. God tells us in Philippians 4:8 to focus on the good. Yet there I was, allowing visions of the task to outweigh the privilege and joy of celebrating people, occasions, and God.

With that somewhat shameful insight, I reflected on what Christmas means. I played Christmas carols and sang along as I unpacked, placed, and hung. I focused on what the decorations represented and the memory each one held. My decorating became a time of worship, grateful remembrance, and elated anticipation. My bah-humbug turned to hallelujah. Yes, our children were coming home, but my approach would have served equally well had they not been.

Over our years we've all commemorated so many birthdays and holidays it's no wonder we sometimes run out of steam. But we can regain it by remembering the essential role we still play in making these celebrations joyous for those who mean the most to us. Even the most reticent people delight in having a fuss made over them, whether they'll admit it or not. As the years pass, every birthday and holiday counts not only as much as ever but even more—for each added year is a privilege not granted to all.

> **Enjoy the little things, for one day you may look back and realize they were the big things.** ROBERT BRAULT

Not every holiday may seem momentous, but what it commemorates is. Each New Year is a time to rejoice in another year lived. If it's been joyful, toot those horns even louder; if it's been tough, give thanks that you have a fresh, untouched year of potential ahead.

On Valentine's Day we focus on the love with which we've been blessed and on those who've brought it to us. Easter, Thanksgiving, and Christmas are opportunities to concentrate on God, his amazing love for us, and his gifts to us. The Fourth of July honors our priceless freedom. Memorial Day recognizes the high price of that freedom and expresses our gratitude for those willing to pay it.

Tradition and decorations are a tribute to what and whom we're celebrating. We can be pivotal in ensuring that not only we but others as well consider these things and praise God, who provides them. Contemplating the object and meaning of our celebration, and thinking of the happiness we're bringing others rather than the work involved, transforms our effort into joy. We have not lost our ability to give others pleasure through our small labors of love.

Dear God,
Thank you for birthdays, holidays, and all celebrations. Thank you most of all for who and what they celebrate. May I not get bogged down in the trappings but enjoy them as a way of enhancing joy and of honoring the person, the event, and you. Remind me to rejoice that I have experienced so many holidays and special occasions, because it means I've been given the gift of years. Keep me from ever taking that treasure for granted. Recharge my energy level. Reignite my enthusiasm. Restore my sense of wonder at what our celebrations commemorate. May my impact always be a positive one. Amen.

SECRET #38

**I have the ability to make celebrations
blah or beautiful.**

39

My Stress Level Matters

I prayed to the LORD, and he answered
me. He freed me from all my fears.

Psalm 34:4

Stress can wreak havoc on our bodies. It can deplete our energy
and give us head and body aches and stomach problems. Stress
can steal our sleep, lower our resistance to illness, injure our relationships, and more.

Jesus asks, "Can all your worries add a single moment to your life?"
(Matthew 6:27). Quite the opposite. When it's long enough or intense enough, stress and worry can kill us. We pay a tremendous price
by worrying. And much of what we worry about never happens. At
this point in our lives, the best thing we can do with what stresses us
is let it go. Excellent advice, but often easier said than done.

> How much pain they have cost us, the evils
> which have never happened! THOMAS JEFFERSON

As Christians, we have an advantage that nonbelievers lack. We
can cast our anxiety, worries, and cares on God, giving them all to
him because he cares about us (1 Peter 5:7). "Give your burdens to
the LORD, and he will take care of you" (Psalm 55:22).

Often I wonder how those who do not know the Lord handle
life's trials. He is "our refuge and strength, an ever-present help in
trouble" (46:1 NIV). Jesus said, "In this world you will have trouble.
But take heart! I have overcome the world" (John 16:33 NIV). It is
only through God that we can overcome the world. We never have
to carry our burdens alone. We can turn them over to God, receiving

in exchange his peace, "which exceeds anything we can understand" (Philippians 4:7).

The Bible contains over two hundred verses telling us to not fear. We can allow stress to cripple us, or we can listen to God as throughout his Word he tells us not to be afraid and to trust him.

> Don't be afraid, for I am with you.
> Don't be discouraged, for I am your God.
> I will strengthen you and help you
> . . . .
> I say to you,
> "Don't be afraid. I am here to help you."
> Isaiah 41:10, 13

I am constantly amazed at how Jesus fills me with his peace when I turn to him. I can be fretting, fuming, stressing, and stewing. But when I take a few deep breaths and ask him for peace, he always gives it to me, usually almost immediately. Peace is a fruit of the Spirit (Galatians 5:22). Ask the Holy Spirit to fill you and produce in you his fruit of peace.

The older we get, the more important it becomes to know that when we feel alone, we are not. He is with us always (Matthew 28:20). He "will keep in perfect peace all who trust in [him], all whose thoughts are fixed on [him]!" (Isaiah 26:3). Let's relax and focus our thoughts on Jesus!

Dear God,
Please quiet my mind and soul. Help me remember that my body feels and manifests all that goes through my mind, and that when my thoughts turn to you, my body will echo your peace. Remind me that my stress level matters, not only to my health but also as a reflection of my trust in you. You have instructed me to not fear or be afraid, because you know the damage that ongoing stress can do. You have offered me the solution—give it all to you. I do that now with praise and thanksgiving. When I feel anxious, stressed, fearful,

or worried, remind me you are right here with me, waiting for and wanting me to hand it all to you. Thank you for the incredible gift that you are always ready to take my burdens, to guide me, and to fill me with your peace. Amen.

SECRET #39

**God will gladly give me his peace
in exchange for my stress.**

40

How I Live Each Day Matters

I have come that they may have
life, and have it to the full.
John 10:10 NIV

When our dogs were with us, one of their favorite treats was a large meat bone. They'd spend hours gnawing it, sucking out its marrow until all that remained was a hollow core. They would have missed a lot of enjoyment (and nourishment) if they had merely licked the surface.

We too will miss out on much of the good God has planned for us if we merely live on life's surface and don't dig deeply into all this life stage can be.

Every day matters, and we matter every day. Each moment, each hour, each day is a piece of our life that will never come again. Each moment, each hour, each day *is* our life.

> **Somebody should tell us, right at the start of our lives, that we are dying. Then we might live life to the limit, every minute of every day. Do it! I say. Whatever you want to do, do it now! There are only so many tomorrows.** ATTRIBUTED TO POPE PAUL VI

Jesus told us he came to give us life to the full. Let's live this gift. Let's soak in and enjoy every moment we have left on this earth. Let's lighten up, give our worries to God, and smile and laugh. Let's dance! And dance we can, at any age, even if only in our minds—and as we dance, let's sing: "Sing to the LORD a new song. Sing his praises. . . . Praise his name with dancing" (Psalm 149:1, 3).

Yes, life—at every age—has its ups and downs, pluses and minuses. So, no need to fret. We can instead put our constant trust in our faithful and loving God. Jesus said, "Don't let your hearts be troubled. Trust in God, and trust also in me" (John 14:1). That is the answer to every question.

Dear God,

May I never disregard the preciousness and brevity of life by letting even one day slip by without appreciation, joy, and the recognition that how I live each twenty-four hours matters—to me, to others, and most importantly, to you. Thank you for the promise you have given in Isaiah 46:4 that even in my old age, you will carry me. As you do, through the ups and the downs, the bright times and the dark times, the victories and the defeats, the joys and the sorrows, through all that this later stage of life brings, help me remember that what I do and who I am each and every day matters. Thank you for helping me know that no matter my age, the answer is YES, I still matter! Amen.

SECRET #40

I can sing and dance, even if only in my mind and heart!

Spread the Word
by Doing One Thing.

- Give a copy of this book as a gift.

- Share the QR code link via your social media.

- Write a review of this book on your blog, favorite bookseller's website, or at ODB.org/store.

- Recommend this book to your church, small group, or book club.

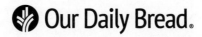

Connect with us. [f] [◎]

Our Daily Bread Publishing
PO Box 3566, Grand Rapids, MI 49501, USA
Email: books@odb.org

Love God. Love Others.

with  Our Daily Bread.

Your gift changes lives.

Connect with us. f ⊙

Our Daily Bread Publishing
PO Box 3566, Grand Rapids, MI 49501, USA
Email: books@odb.org

How do you deepen your relationship with and understanding of God?

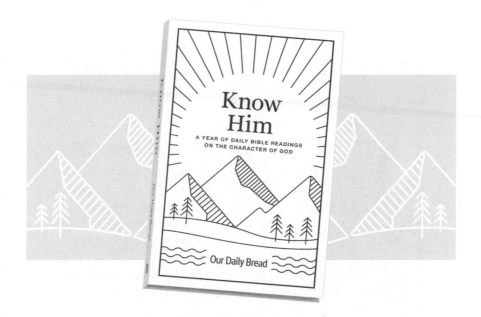

At the source.
Get to know Him through His own Word, the Bible.

Know Him devotes 365 days to revealing the character of God solely through Scripture. These passages, drawn from every book of the Bible, highlight 12 unchanging attributes of our Creator. Whether you're new to the Bible or a longtime reader, you'll gain a deeper awe of God's holiness, transcendence, and glory along with a renewed appreciation for His mercy, justice, and truth.

Buy it today

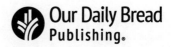

Timeless Wisdom to Inspire Your Faith

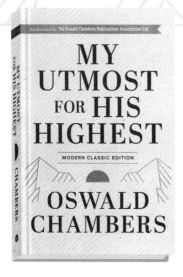

Modern Classic Edition, 2023:

- NIV Bible translation
- Preserved the original language and context, maintaining Chambers's message and voice, while bringing clarity and readability
- Adapted from the Classic by journalist Macy Halford

ISBN 1640702555

Updated Edition, 1992:

- NKJV Bible translation
- Translated for modern readers for accurate and readable edition
- Researched and edited by Rev. James Reimann

ISBN 1627078762

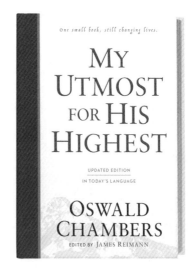

Classic Edition, 1935:

- KJV Bible translation
- Oswald's word-for-word original text
- Compiled by Oswald's wife, Gertrude "Biddy" Chambers

ISBN 1627078788

Order yours today

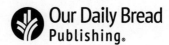